INTERVENTIONAL CARDIOLOGY CLINICS

www.interventional.theclinics.com

Editor-in-Chief

MATTHEW J. PRICE

Transcatheter Tricuspid Valve Intervention

Interventional Therapy for Pulmonary Embolism

January 2018 • Volume 7 • Number 1

Editors

AZEEM LATIB
JAY GIRI

ELSEVIER

1600 John F. Kennedy Boulevard • Suite 1800 • Philadelphia, Pennsylvania, 19103-2899

http://www.theclinics.com

INTERVENTIONAL CARDIOLOGY CLINICS Volume 7, Number 1
January 2018 ISSN 2211-7458, ISBN-13: 978-0-323-57061-9

Editor: Lauren Boyle
Developmental Editor: Donald Mumford

Interventional Cardiology Clinics (ISSN 2211-7458) is published quarterly by Elsevier Inc., 360 Park Avenue South, New York, NY 10010-1710. Months of issue are January, April, July, and October. Subscription prices are USD 195 per year for US individuals, USD 449 for US institutions, USD 100 per year for US students, USD 195 per year for Canadian individuals, USD 536 for Canadian institutions, USD 150 per year for Canadian students, USD 295 per year for international individuals, USD 536 for international institutions, and USD 150 per year for international students. To receive student/resident rate, orders must be accompanied by name of affiliated institution, date of term, and the *signature* of program/residency coordinator on institution letterhead. Orders will be billed at individual rate until proof of status is received. Foreign air speed delivery is included in all *Clinics* subscription prices. All prices are subject to change without notice. **POSTMASTER:** Send address changes to *Interventional Cardiology Clinics*, Elsevier Health Sciences Division, Subscription Customer Service, 3251 Riverport Lane, Maryland Heights, MO 63043. **Customer Service: Telephone: 1-800-654-2452** (U.S. and Canada); **1-314-447-8871** (outside U.S. and Canada). **Fax: 1-314-447-8029. E-mail: journalscustomerservice-usa@elsevier.com (for print support); journalsonlinesupport-usa@elsevier.com (for online support).**

Reprints. For copies of 100 or more of articles in this publication, please contact the Commercial Reprints Department, Elsevier Inc., 360 Park Avenue South, New York, NY 10010-1710. Tel.: 212-633-3874; Fax: 212-633-3820; E-mail: reprints@elsevier.com.

CONTRIBUTORS

EDITOR-IN-CHIEF

MATTHEW J. PRICE, MD
Director, Cardiac Catheterization Laboratory,
Division of Cardiovascular Diseases, Scripps
Clinic, Assistant Professor, Scripps
Translational Science Institute, La Jolla,
California, USA

EDITORS

AZEEM LATIB, MD, FESC, FACC
Interventional Cardiology Unit, San Raffaele
Scientific Institute, EMO GVM Centro Cuore
Columbus, Milan, Italy

JAY GIRI, MD, MPH
Assistant Professor, Director, Peripheral
Intervention, Associate Director, Penn
Cardiovascular Outcomes, Quality, and
Evaluative Research Center, Interventional
Cardiology and Vascular Medicine, Division of
Cardiovascular Medicine, Perelman School of
Medicine University of Pennsylvania,
Philadelphia, Pennsylvania, USA

AUTHORS

EUSTACHIO AGRICOLA, MD
Director, Echocardiography Laboratory,
Clinical Cardiology Unit, San Raffaele
Scientific Institute, Milan, Italy

FRANCESCO ANCONA, MD
Echocardiography Laboratory, Clinical
Cardiology Unit, San Raffaele Scientific
Institute, Milan, Italy

LAWRENCE ANG, MD
Division of Cardiovascular Medicine, Sulpizio
Cardiovascular Center, UC San Diego,
La Jolla, California, USA

CHIRAG BAVISHI, MD, MPH
Mount Sinai St Luke's-Roosevelt Hospital
Center, New York, New York, USA

OMID BEHNAMFAR, MD
Division of Cardiovascular Medicine, Sulpizio
Cardiovascular Center, UC San Diego,
La Jolla, California, USA

NIMROD BLANK, MD
Department of Medicine, Detroit Medical
Center, Wayne State University, Detroit,
Michigan, USA

NICOLA BUZZATTI, MD
Cardiac Surgery Department, San Raffaele
Scientific Institute, Milan, Italy

CRISTINA CAPOGROSSO, MD
Echocardiography Laboratory, Clinical
Cardiology Unit, San Raffaele Scientific
Institute, Milan, Italy

SANJAY CHATTERJEE, MD
Consultant, Apollo Gleneagles Hospital,
Kolkata, India

SAURAV CHATTERJEE, MD
Attending Interventional Cardiologist, The
Hoffman Heart and Vascular Institute, Saint
Francis Hospital, Teaching Affiliate, University
of Connecticut School of Medicine, Hartford,
Connecticut, USA

MICHELE DE BONIS, MD
Cardiac Surgery Department, San Raffaele
Scientific Institute, Milan, Italy

HENRYK DREGER, MD
Department of Cardiology,
Charité – Universitaetsmedizin Berlin, German
Centre for Cardiovascular Research (DZHK),
University Heart Center, Berlin, Germany

MAHIR ELDER, MD
Professor, Department of Medicine, Detroit
Medical Center, Wayne State University,
Detroit, Michigan, USA

HANS R. FIGULLA, MD
University Heart Center Jena, Jena, Germany

JAY GIRI, MD, MPH
Assistant Professor, Director, Peripheral
Intervention, Associate Director, Penn
Cardiovascular Outcomes, Quality and
Evaluative Research Center, Interventional
Cardiology and Vascular Medicine, Division of
Cardiovascular Medicine, Perelman School of
Medicine University of Pennsylvania,
Philadelphia, Pennsylvania, USA

REBECCA T. HAHN, MD
Director of Interventional Echocardiography,
Columbia University Medical Center,
New York Presbyterian Hospital, New York,
New York, USA

WISSAM A. JABER, MD
Division of Cardiology, Emory University
School of Medicine, Atlanta, Georgia, USA

AMIR KAKI, MD
Associate Professor, Department of Medicine,
Detroit Medical Center, Wayne State
University, Detroit, Michigan, USA

SAMIR R. KAPADIA, MD
Section Head, Interventional Cardiology,
Director, Sones Cardiac Catheterization
Laboratory, Heart & Vascular Institute,
Cleveland Clinic, Cleveland, Ohio, USA

JOHN ANDREW KAUFMAN, MD, MS
Chairman, Department of Interventional
Radiology, Director, Dotter Interventional
Institute, Frederick S. Keller Chair of
Interventional Radiology, Oregon Health &
Science University, Portland, Oregon, USA

NICK H. KIM, MD
Division of Pulmonary and Critical Care
Medicine, Sulpizio Cardiovascular Center, UC
San Diego, La Jolla, California, USA

AMAR KRISHNASWAMY, MD
Program Director, Interventional Cardiology
Fellowship, Section of Interventional
Cardiology, Department of Cardiovascular
Medicine, Heart & Vascular Institute,
Cleveland Clinic, Cleveland, Ohio, USA

AZEEM LATIB, MD, FESC, FACC
Interventional Cardiology Unit, San Raffaele
Scientific Institute, EMO GVM Centro Cuore
Columbus, Milan, Italy

MICHAEL LAULE, MD
Department of Cardiology,
Charité – Universitaetsmedizin Berlin, German
Centre for Cardiovascular Research (DZHK),
University Heart Center, Berlin, Germany

ALEXANDER LAUTEN, MD
Department of Cardiology,
Charité – Universitaetsmedizin Berlin,
German Centre for Cardiovascular Research
(DZHK), University Heart Center, Berlin,
Germany

SCOTT LIM, MD
Department of Cardiology, University of
Virginia, Charlottesville, Virginia, USA

EHTISHAM MAHMUD, MD, FACC, FSCAI
Division of Cardiovascular Medicine, Sulpizio
Cardiovascular Center, UC San Diego,
La Jolla, California, USA

ANTONIO MANGIERI, MD
Interventional Cardiology Unit, San Raffaele
Scientific Institute, Milan, Italy

ALBERTO MARGONATO, MD
Echocardiography Laboratory, Clinical
Cardiology Unit, San Raffaele Scientific
Institute, Milan, Italy

CLAUDIA MARINI, MD
Echocardiography Laboratory, Clinical
Cardiology Unit, San Raffaele Scientific
Institute, Milan, Italy

MICHAEL C. McDANIEL, MD
Division of Cardiology, Emory University
School of Medicine, Atlanta, Georgia, USA

NEIL MOAT, MD
Cardiac Surgery Department, Royal Brompton
& Harefield NHS Foundation Trust, London,
United Kingdom

TAMAM MOHAMAD, MD
Associate Professor, Department of Medicine,
Detroit Medical Center, Wayne State
University, Detroit, Michigan, USA

JOSE NAVIA, MD
Department of Cardiothoracic Surgery, Heart
& Vascular Institute, Cleveland Clinic,
Cleveland, Ohio, USA

MOHIT PAHUJA, MD
Department of Medicine, Detroit Medical
Center, Wayne State University, Detroit,
Michigan, USA

MITUL P. PATEL, MD
Division of Cardiovascular Medicine, Sulpizio
Cardiovascular Center, UC San Diego,
La Jolla, California, USA

DAVID POCH, MD
Division of Pulmonary and Critical Care
Medicine, Sulpizio Cardiovascular Center,
UC San Diego, La Jolla, California, USA

RISHI PURI, MBBS, PhD
Quebec Heart and Lung Institute, Laval
University, Quebec City, Quebec, Canada

JOSEP RODÉS-CABAU, MD
Quebec Heart and Lung Institute, Laval
University, Quebec City, Quebec, Canada

JASON H. ROGERS, MD
Division of Cardiovascular Medicine, UC Davis
Medical Center, Sacramento, California, USA

PARTHA SARDAR, MD
Division of Cardiovascular Medicine, The
University of Utah, Salt Lake City, Utah, USA

THEODORE SCHREIBER, MD
Professor, Department of Medicine, Detroit
Medical Center, Wayne State University,
Detroit, Michigan, USA

ADI SHEMESH, MD
Department of Medicine, Detroit Medical
Center, Wayne State University, Detroit,
Michigan, USA

AKHILESH K. SISTA, MD
Section Chief, Vascular and Interventional
Radiology, Department of Radiology, NYU
Langone Medical Center, New York, New
York, USA

KARL STANGL, MD
Department of Cardiology,
Charité – Universitaetsmedizin Berlin, German
Centre for Cardiovascular Research (DZHK),
University Heart Center, Berlin, Germany

STEFANO STELLA, MD
Echocardiography Laboratory, Clinical
Cardiology Unit, San Raffaele Scientific
Institute, Milan, Italy

GILBERT H.L. TANG, MD, MSc, MBA
Surgical Director, Structural Heart Program,
Department of Cardiovascular Surgery, Mount
Sinai Health System, New York, New York, USA

BEDROS TASLAKIAN, MD
Clinical Fellow, Vascular and Interventional
Radiology, Department of Radiology,
NYU Langone Medical Center, New York,
New York, USA

HAFEEZ UL HASSAN VIRK, MD
Mount Sinai St Luke's-Roosevelt Hospital
Center, New York, New York, USA

CONTENTS

Section 1: Transcatheter Tricuspid Valve Intervention

The tricuspid valve is a complex dynamic apparatus made up of many different closely linked structures: the annulus, the three leaflets, the chordae, the papillary muscles, and the right ventricle. Other nearby structures, such as the coronary sinus ostium, the conduction system, the membranous septum, and the right coronary artery must be taken into account when dealing with the tricuspid. Annulus dilation and leaflet tethering due to right ventricular remodeling are the 2 major mechanisms responsible for most tricuspid regurgitation cases. Precise knowledge of tricuspid anatomy and function, as well as careful preoperative planning, is fundamental for successful transcatheter tricuspid procedures.

Nowadays, reasonable transcatheter tricuspid valve (TV) interventions are emerging as therapeutic options for functional tricuspid regurgitation (TR). The preprocedural planning is based on a multimodal imaging approach, which aims to (1) define the mechanisms of TR, (2) characterize TV morphology, (3) analyze the anatomic relationship between the TV apparatus and other structures, and (4) determine the size of the tricuspid annulus and vena cavae. Intraprocedural guidance is based mainly on transesophageal echocardiography (seldom transthoracic) and fluoroscopy, with the recent introduction of fusion imaging.

The tricuspid valve was ignored for a long time. The prevalence of severe tricuspid regurgitation is not negligible, however, and is associated with poor prognosis. In cases of primary tricuspid regurgitation, surgical options are limited by a high risk of mortality and morbidity. New percutaneous approaches are becoming available to meet this consistent unmet clinical need. This article presents the current available devices that reproduce both the complete and uncomplete surgical annuloplasty techniques.

Symptomatic severe tricuspid regurgitation (TR), if untreated, carries a dismal prognosis. These patients are at very high risk for surgical repair or replacement, and transcatheter options to treat TR are emerging. More than 300 transcatheter tricuspid repairs with the MitraClip system have been performed worldwide with promising results. The TriClip system, with the MitraClip NT delivered via a dedicated tricuspid steerable guide catheter, is under investigation. This article describes the step-by-step technique on using the MitraClip system to perform transcatheter tricuspid repair using echocardiographic and fluoroscopic guidance. The latest data on worldwide experience with tricuspid clipping are also discussed.

Significant tricuspid valve disease affects many patients with left-sided heart disease. Concomitant tricuspid valve surgery for at least moderate tricuspid insufficiency is undertaken far less frequently at the time of left-sided heart surgery. The
burden of residual tricuspid disease in high-surgical-risk patients has spawned
the evolution of several percutaneous treatment options. A dedicated percutaneously delivered tricuspid spacer device (FORMA Repair System) has been
developed and trialed in humans. This system anchors a spacer to reduce the
regurgitant orifice area, thereby providing a surface for valve leaflet coaptation.
This article provides an overview of the FORMA Repair System to date.

Transcatheter therapy has expanded the treatment options for patients with
heart valve disease. With the growing understanding of tricuspid regurgitation
and its natural history, it becomes increasingly obvious that this patient population is a heterogeneous cohort presenting for treatment in different stages of
a continuous disease process. It is still unclear which interventional approach
will result in functional and clinical success and in which subtype of patient population. This article reviews the pathophysiologic background and current evidence for caval valve implantation and examines the potential role of this
approach for the treatment of severe tricuspid regurgitation.

Tricuspid regurgitation (TR) is a common entity, most commonly functional in
nature due to right-sided dysfunction in the setting of concomitant cardiac disease or pulmonary hypertension. Patients living with TR often experience
numerous limitations as a result of right-sided heart failure symptoms,
including functional decline, frequent hospitalizations, liver failure, and kidney
failure. Furthermore, patients with significant TR demonstrate worse survival,
although a cause-and-effect relationship has not been proven. For patients
with a degenerated surgical bioprosthesis or valve ring, placement of a transcatheter aortic valve prosthesis in a valve-in-valve or valve-in-ring fashion may
provide symptomatic benefit. For patients with native valve regurgitation, novel
devices for treatment are under development.

Section 2: Interventional Therapy for Pulmonary Embolism

Acute pulmonary embolism presents a clinical challenge for optimal risk stratification. Although this condition is associated with significant morbidity and mortality at the population level, the spectrum of presentation in an individual patient
varies from mild symptoms to cardiac arrest. Treatment options include anticoagulation, systemic thrombolysis, catheter-based interventions, and surgical embolectomy. In this article, an attempt is made to optimally identify patients who,
based on available evidence, may benefit from systemic thrombolytic therapy.
The clinical efficacy of systemic thrombolysis must be balanced against increased
risks of major bleeding and intracranial hemorrhage.

Acute pulmonary embolism (PE) is the third most common cause of death among hospitalized patients. Treatment escalation beyond anticoagulation therapy is necessary in patients with cardiogenic shock and may be of benefit in select normotensive patients with right-sided heart strain. Percutaneous catheter-based techniques (catheter-directed mechanical thrombectomy, clot maceration, and/or pharmacologic thrombolysis) as an alternative or adjunct to systemic thrombolysis can rapidly debulk central clot in patients with shock. Catheter-directed thrombolysis, which uses a low-dose intraclot prolonged thrombolytic infusion, is a promising but insufficiently studied therapy for patients presenting with acute intermediate-risk PE.

A significant number of patients with high-risk pulmonary embolism have contraindications to thrombolytic therapy. Catheter-based therapy may be helpful and consists of a multitude of catheters and techniques, some old and some new. Although there are few data supporting the use of any of these techniques, there has been a recent rise in interest and use of catheter-based pulmonary embolectomy. This article describes the contemporary devices used in pulmonary embolism treatment, discusses their challenges, and proposes some future directions.

Chronic thromboembolic pulmonary hypertension (CTEPH) is associated with several risk factors but is most frequently seen as a rare consequence of an acute pulmonary embolism. Surgical pulmonary thromboendarterectomy (PTE) is potentially curative for CTEPH, with the best outcomes seen for the treatment of primarily proximal, accessible lobar or segmental disease. For surgically inoperable patients, percutaneous balloon pulmonary angioplasty (BPA) is feasible and has good short- to mid-term efficacy outcomes. This article focuses on the technique and outcomes associated with BPA, which has emerged as a new therapeutic option for CTEPH.

Temporary mechanical circulatory support (MCS) devices have a role in treating high-risk patients with pulmonary embolism with cardiogenic shock. Mechanical circulatory device selection should be made based on center experience and device-specific features. All current devices are effective in decreasing right arterial pressure and providing circulatory support of 4 to 5 L/min. The pulmonary artery pulsatility index may prove to be an unreliable method to assess right ventricular function. Careful clinical evaluation on an individual patient basis should determine the need for MCS.

The inferior vena cava filter clinical environment is notable for the degree of controversy, uncertainty, and fear associated with these devices by both physicians and the public. This article reviews some of the more important current issues with these devices, as well as emerging and future trends.

TRANSCATHETER TRICUSPID VALVE INTERVENTION/INTERVENTIONAL THERAPY FOR PULMONARY EMBOLISM

THE CLINICS ARE NOW AVAILABLE ONLINE!

Access your subscription at:
www.theclinics.com

PREFACE

Transcatheter Tricuspid Valve Intervention: Addressing an Unmet Clinical Need

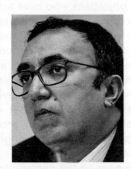

Azeem Latib, MD, FESC, FACC
Editor

Functional tricuspid regurgitation (FTR) is the most common manifestation of tricuspid valve disease and is caused by left-sided heart disease or pulmonary disease in most cases, but in some cases, can also be isolated due to chronic atrial fibrillation. FTR has traditionally been considered a benign valvulopathy that resolves with treatment of left-sided disease and that can be adequately treated with diuretics. Indeed, in many patients with FTR undergoing left-sided surgery, the tricuspid valve is not repaired due to underestimation of the severity of tricuspid regurgitation (TR) in the operating room, unjustified concerns that tricuspid repair increases surgical risk, or a belief that the TR will resolve. However, in recent years, we have gained a better understanding of the prognostic significance and natural history of TR. FTR has been shown to be an independent predictor of mortality in every surgical, percutaneous, or heart failure population in which it has been studied, irrespective of left ventricular function, right ventricular function, or pulmonary hypertension. The importance of annular dilatation has also become evident because the severity of TR fluctuates, is volume dependent, and can be modified with diuretic therapy. However, once the tricuspid annulus is dilated, FTR recurs after left-sided surgery and progresses irrespective of diuretic

therapy. It has also become apparent that the majority of patients with severe, symptomatic FTR are not referred for intervention because the only treatment that has been available is surgical repair or replacement, which is often associated with an unacceptably high morbidity and mortality due to the multiple comorbidities in these patients and because as many as two-thirds are redo cardiac surgery patients. This is also compounded by the fact that most patients with severe TR are asymptomatic or have minimal and vague symptoms for long periods before eventually developing right-sided heart failure. They are usually only referred when heart failure symptoms are no longer responsive to diuretic therapy. At this stage, the valve is often severely remodeled; severe right ventricular dysfunction is present, and patients may have multiple comorbidities (especially renal and hepatic dysfunction) and are now not only inoperable but also poor candidates for less-invasive therapies. As a result, FTR has been identified as an important unmet clinical need requiring less invasive therapies, and numerous transcatheter therapies have been developed in an attempt to address this valvulopathy.

The tricuspid valve has been relatively ignored by the cardiology community, and thus, the anatomy, pathophysiology, natural history, and

Intervent Cardiol Clin 7 (2018) xiii–xiv
https://doi.org/10.1016/j.iccl.2017.10.001
2211-7458/18/© 2017 Published by Elsevier Inc.

imaging are not well defined. Although an atrio-ventricular valve, the tricuspid valve has important differences as compared with the mitral valve, including 3 leaflets, annular and leaflet tissue appears more fragile, close proximity of the right coronary artery and atrioventricular node, and a large heterogeneity of the patient subsets with secondary TR. A thorough understanding of the anatomy is needed if we are to be successful in percutaneously treating the tricuspid valve. The main mechanisms of FTR are annular dilatation with leaflet tethering playing an important part in more advanced stages of FTR. Thus, a number of transcatheter devices have been developed to correct these mechanisms either by annuloplasty to reduce annular dimensions, leaflet devices to increase leaflet coaptation, heterotopic valve implantation to decrease the negative effects of caval backflow, or even transcatheter tricuspid valve replacement, which may be an important solution in patients with advanced valvular remodeling. All these devices are in preclinical, early feasibility, or first-in-man evaluation with the objective of evaluating the feasibility and safety of these devices. As regards evaluating efficacy, the biggest challenge is that we are currently evaluating these devices in patients with advanced tricuspid valve disease with torrential TR, where complete elimination of the TR is impossible. Despite this, an interesting finding has been that even modest reductions of TR have resulted in significant improvements in symptoms and quality of life.

As this is a rapidly evolving field, in this issue of *Interventional Cardiology Clinics*, we have assembled some of the leading experts in the world to share their experiences and provide the reader with an up-to-date overview of this innovative subject. This issue begins with a surgeon's perspective of the anatomy of the tricuspid valve complex followed by a detailed and systematic approach to the standardized echocardiographic imaging of the tricuspid valve, which is essential to guide transcatheter interventions. Both of these articles are essential to the understanding of the mechanisms and challenges of the different percutaneous options that are available. The issue continues with a detailed review (device overview, procedural steps, and available clinical data) of the available devices by physicians who have actually performed these procedures. It is important for the reader to keep in mind when reading these device reviews that the current clinical experience is still very limited; there are no standardized and uniform definitions for evaluating efficacy of transcatheter tricuspid intervention, and thus device comparison is not possible; and finally, that we are currently treating patients with very advanced disease in whom it may sometimes be challenging to demonstrate the benefits of reducing TR.

Our sincere gratitude goes to the contributors of this issue, and we hope that this exceptional collection of articles will not only be educational but also raise awareness of this important clinical problem, the potential innovative therapies that are becoming available, and thus, eventually lead to the earlier treatment of patients with FTR.

Azeem Latib, MD, FESC, FACC
Interventional Cardiology Unit
San Raffaele Scientific Institute
Via Olgettina 60, Milan 20132, Italy

Interventional Cardiology Unit
EMO-GVM Centro Cuore Columbus
Milan, Italy

E-mail address:
alatib@gmail.com

Section 1: Transcatheter Tricuspid Valve Intervention

Anatomy of the Tricuspid Valve, Pathophysiology of Functional Tricuspid Regurgitation, and Implications for Percutaneous Therapies

Nicola Buzzatti, MD[a],*, Michele De Bonis, MD[a],
Neil Moat, MD[b]

KEYWORDS

- Tricuspid • Right ventricle • Transcatheter • Anatomy • Functional

KEY POINTS

- The tricuspid valve is a complex dynamic structure whose function depends on the harmony of several different components: annulus, leaflets, chordae, papillary muscles, and right ventricle.
- Several nonvalvular structures, such as the coronary sinus ostium, the conduction system, the membranous septum, and the right coronary artery are in close relationship with the tricuspid annulus.
- Annulus dilation and leaflet tethering due to right ventricle remodeling are the 2 major pathophysiologic mechanisms behind functional tricuspid regurgitation.
- Precise knowledge of tricuspid anatomy and function as well as careful preoperative planning is fundamental for the development of transcatheter tricuspid interventions.

Over the past few years, the development of transcatheter technologies allowed for the introduction of complex percutaneous procedures, such as prostheses implantation and valve repair, for the treatment of valvular heart diseases.[1,2] Although today the application of transcatheter technologies in their early phase of development is mostly limited to selected inoperable and high-risk patients, wide expansion to lower-risk patients can be anticipated in the future. Following the aortic valve and the mitral valve, the tricuspid valve is receiving increasing attention from the interventional cardiology community.[3]

The tricuspid atrioventricular (AV) valve separates the right atrium (RA) from the right ventricle (RV), controlling blood flow between them. Similar to the mitral valve, it is actually a complex apparatus whose function depends on the harmony of several different structures, closely linked to each other. The tricuspid valve anatomy, however, shows greater variability than the anatomy of the mitral valve. Close to the valve itself, other important surrounding structures, although not strictly valvular components, can be useful anatomic markers and need to be taken into consideration to avoid complications whenever the tricuspid valve apparatus is addressed by an intervention.

ANATOMY

Gross anatomy of the tricuspid valve and of the right heart is depicted in **Figs. 1** and **2**.

Disclosure Statement: The authors have nothing to disclose.
[a] Cardiac Surgery Department, San Raffaele Scientific Institute, Via Olgettina 60, Milan 20129, Italy; [b] Cardiac Surgery Department, Royal Brompton & Harefield Trust, Sydney Street, London SW3 6NP, UK
* Corresponding author.
E-mail address: buzzatti.nicola@hsr.it

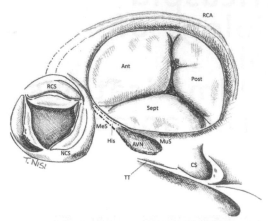

Fig. 1. Schematic representation of the surgical view of the tricuspid valve from the RA. Ant, anterior leaflet; AVN, AV node; CS, coronary sinus ostium; His, bundle of His; MeS, septum membranosum; MuS, muscular portion of the AV septum; NCS, noncoronary sinus of the aorta; Post, posterior leaflet; RCS, right coronary sinus of the aorta; Sept, septal leaflet; TT, tendon of Todaro.

The Tricuspid Apparatus

Historically, autopsy and open heart surgery have been the primary sources of anatomic knowledge on the tricuspid valve. With the development of ultrasound technology, 2-D/3-D echocardiography has become the most frequently used method to study the tricuspid and RV anatomy, thanks to its easy accessibility and ability to provide concomitant functional assessment. More recently, CT has been increasingly adopted to evaluate the anatomy of mitral and tricuspid valves in patients screened for new transcatheter technologies.[4] The principal advantages of CT are its high anatomic spatial resolution, its user-friendly multiplanar and 3-D interface, and the ability to simulate device positioning inside a patient's heart. CT assessment of the tricuspid is, however, challenging and still evolving.[5] Finally, MRI is currently the gold standard for the assessment of RV morphology and function and it may be useful in functional evaluation of the tricuspid valve in cases of poor echocardiographic imaging quality.[4] Nevertheless its use in real-word daily practice is still limited.

The tricuspid is the most anterior (close to the chest wall and far from the esophagus) of all the heart valves. Its orientation within the normal heart is nearly vertical. The orifice of the normal tricuspid valve has an approximately oval shape, and it is larger than that of the mitral valve. Based on autopsy, the normal tricuspid orifice in the adult approximates a diameter of 20 mm/m^2 and an area of 5.8 cm^2/m^2.[6] The tricuspid annulus is relatively indistinct, especially in the septal region. When evaluated by echocardiography, the healthy annulus is a nonplanar structure with an elliptical pattern that can change markedly with loading conditions.[7,8] Posteroseptal and anterolateral segments of the annulus are closer to the RV apex, the lowest point being the posteroseptal segment near the coronary sinus. In contrast, anteroseptal and posterolateral segments are higher (toward the RA), the highest point in the anteroseptal segment, near the RV outflow tract and aortic valve. Physiologically the normal annulus moves up away from and down towards the RV apex within the cardiac cycle. Normal tricuspid annular plane systolic excursion (TAPSE) along the longitudinal axis of the RV, as assessed by echocardiography, is greater than or equal to 16 mm.[9] Tricuspid orifice increases its size from midsystole to early diastole, decreases during mid-diastole, and increases again in late diastole at the time of atrial contraction. The normal excursion of tricuspid area is 25% to 30%. Echocardiographic normal tricuspid valve actual diameter in adults is 28 mm ± 5 mm in the 4-chamber view and actual valve area is 11 cm^2 ± 2 cm^2.[10,11] 2-D echo is known to underestimate actual tricuspid annulus size compared with 3-D echo. Recent CT data report a maximum diastolic area of 10.7 cm^2 ± 2.2 cm^2 in healthy persons.[12]

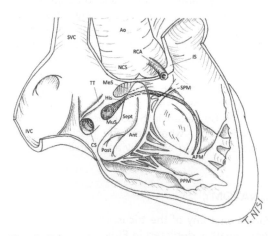

Fig. 2. Schematic representation of the RA, tricuspid valve and RV. Ant, anterior leaflet; Ao, aorta; APM, anterior papillary muscles; AVN, AV node; CS, coronary sinus ostium; His, bundle of His; IS, infundibular septum; IVC, inferior vena cava; MeS, septum membranosum; MuS, muscular portion of the AV septum; NCS, noncoronary sinus of the aorta; Post, posterior leaflet; PPM, posterior papillary muscle; Sept, septal leaflet; SPM, septal papillary muscle; SVC, superior vena cava; TT, tendon of Todaro.

The leaflets and chordae tendineae are thinner than those of the mitral valve. The tricuspid valve has 3 leaflets unequal in size: anterior, posterior, and septal. The anterior leaflet is the biggest of the 3 leaflets and may have notches creating subdivisions.[13] Its chordae tendineae arise from anterior and medial papillary muscles. The posterior leaflet is usually the smallest and is commonly scalloped; its chordae originate from the posterior and anterior papillary muscles; it is attached wholly to the ventricular free wall. The septal leaflet is usually slightly larger than the posterior leaflet. Its chordae arise from the posterior and septal papillary muscles; most of this leaflet and its chordae attach to the membranous and muscular portions of the ventricular septum. In a normal heart, the tricuspid valve is located slightly closer to the apex than the mitral valve. The space in between the septal insertion of the tricuspid valve and the septal insertion of the anterior leaflet of mitral valve belongs to the membranous septum that separates the left ventricle from the RA. Tricuspid leaflets are easily visualized by echocardiography and not as easily by CT scan.

Marked variability of papillary muscle anatomy is characteristic of the tricuspid valve. Usually 2 or 3 papillary muscles can be seen. The anterior is the most prominent, its base arising from the right ventricular free wall and trabecula septomarginalis. The posterior is often bifid or trifid. The septal (medial or muscle of Lancisi) papillary muscle is the least prominent and sometimes can be even absent, with the multiple chordal attachments arising directly from the ventricular wall. The right bundle branch courses just below it.

The RV has a complex shape, normally triangular when viewed longitudinally and crescent-shaped when viewed transversally. The RV is divided into 3 portions: inlet, containing tricuspid valve and surrounding ventricular septum; sinus, or coarse trabecular portion; and outlet, or conus portion, containing infundibular septum and pulmonary valve. The infundibular septum separates the pulmonary from the aortic and tricuspid valves. A right/lateral extension of infundibular septum merges with RV as ventriculo-infundibular fold (parietal band). Medially and to the left, infundibular septum merges with RV to form a Y-shaped muscle bundle called the trabecula septomarginalis (septal band). The trabecula septomarginalis extends to the apex as the moderator band. The inlet and outlet valves of the RV are thus widely separated. The entire sinus portion of the RV and most of the infundibulum (both free wall and septum) are trabeculated. Its complex shape is difficult to model geometrically as opposed to the left ventricle, which explains some of the difficulties in assessing right ventricular volumes and function by echocardiography.

Surrounding Structures

The ostium of the coronary sinus lies superiorly and medially to the orifice of the inferior vena cava in the RA, between this orifice and the septal portion of the tricuspid annulus. It is an important anatomic land mark defining the base of the triangle of Koch. Moreover, the posteroseptal commissure is usually located just close to its lateral edge.

As a result of the low (apical) position of the septal leaflet, which is lower than the mitral annulus (especially posteriorly), the AV septum is created. This separates the RA from the left ventricle. It consists of a superior membranous portion and an inferior muscular portion.

The membranous septum is the fibrous part of the cardiac septum separating the left ventricular outflow tract from, in part, the RV and, in part, the RA. The line of division between these components is determined by attachment of the tricuspid valve annulus to the septum. The membranous septum usually lies beneath the septal leaflet inferior to the anteroseptal commissure, but attachments at the septal and anterior leaflets are variable, so parts of either may attach to the membranous septum. The membranous septum is easily recognizable on CT images.

The AV node lies directly on the RA side of the central fibrous body (right trigone) in the muscular portion of the AV septum, just anterosuperior to the ostium of the coronary sinus.[14,15] It has a flattened oblong shape and an average dimension in adults of 1 mm × 3 mm × 6 mm. Its left surface lies against the medial aspect of the mitral annulus. Viewed from the RA, the AV node can be localized within the triangle of Koch, formed by the tricuspid annulus, tendon of Todaro (a continuation of the eustachian valve that runs to the central fibrous body), and coronary sinus ostium. The common AV bundle (bundle of His) is a direct continuation of the AV node. The bundle descends through the right-sided part of the right trigone of the central fibrous body to reach the posteroinferior margin of the membranous ventricular septum. This area is just inferior to the commissure between the tricuspid valve's septal and anterior leaflets, usually approximately 5 mm inferior to the commissure. The diameter of the bundle at the central fibrous body is approximately 1 mm. The bundle runs along the posteroinferior border of the membranous septum and crest of the muscular ventricular septum, giving off fibers that form the left bundle branch. This branching occurs beneath the commissure between the right and noncoronary cusps of the aortic valve, over a distance of 6.5 mm to 20 mm, after which the remaining fibers form the right bundle branch. The bundle of His lies on the left side of the ventricular septal crest in approximately 75% to 80% of human hearts and on the right side of the crest in the remainder.

The right coronary artery (RCA) courses down the right AV groove close to the tricuspid annulus. Branches supplying the anterior right ventricular free wall exit from the AV sulcus in a looping fashion because of the depth of the RCA in the sulcus. The relationship between RCA and the tricuspid valve is subject to great variability. A study on 44 normal human hearts found that the RCA approximated to the tricuspid annulus at the level of the superoanterior (median distance from the nearest adjacent RCA to the endocardium 3.9 mm, range 2.3 mm–8.2 mm) to anterior (median 6.8 mm, range 5.9 mm–11.0 mm) segments and traversed alongside the annulus until it reached the cardiac crux. Accordingly, the distance between endocardium and RCA gradually decreased and became less than 3 mm at the posterior aspect (median 2.1; range 2.0–4.0 mm; $P<.001$ both in superoanterior vs inferior segments and in anterior vs inferior segments).[16] A CT analysis of 250 patients also reported a mean distance of RCA to anterior leaflet of 8.8 mm ± 4.5 mm and to posterior leaflet of 3.6 mm ± 3.4 mm.[17] Maximal distance to the RCA less than or equal to 2 mm was found at the level of anterior leaflet in 7.4% cases but at the level of posterior leaflet in 31.5% of patients. In this series, the RCA coursed at the same level of anterior and posterior leaflets in 64.8% of patients, while remaining superior in 10.4%, and crossed the annulus in 24.8% of patients. In a subgroup of patients affected by TR, the RCA never remained superior to the annulus level.

Superior and inferior venae cavae bring back deoxygenated blood from the body to the RA. They are thin-walled, compliant, and easily compressible. The superior vena cava extends for a distance of 6 cm to 8 cm; the azygos vein is its only major venous channel, entering posteriorly just above the pericardial reflection. The inferior vena cava is formed by the confluence of the 2 common iliac veins at the L5 vertebral level. It runs retroperitoneal along the right side of the vertebral column with the aorta lying laterally on the left. It passes through the diaphragm at the caval hiatus at the T8 level and has a short intrathoracic course. Its orifice in the RA, approximately 30 mm in diameter, is inferior and lateral to the tricuspid annulus. Observed distance between junction with RA and the first hepatic vein at CT was reported as 14.1 mm ± 5.1 mm.[17]

PATHOPHYSIOLOGY OF FUNCTIONAL TRICUSPID REGURGITATION

Tricuspid regurgitation (TR) is known to be associated with increased morbidity and mortality.[18,19] There are many different etiologies of TR. Functional TR (fTR) is currently the most common form of TR in Western countries.[20] fTR is a continuum and a dynamic process, extremely dependent on heart loading conditions.

Functional Tricuspid Regurgitation Mechanisms

Annular dilation and leaflet tethering are the 2 fundamental pathophysiologic mechanisms ultimately responsible for fTR.[21,22]

Annular dilation develops laterally along the RV free wall, both in anterior and posterior directions (Fig. 3). The annulus loses its 3-D shape, becoming more circular and flat (Fig. 4).[8,22,23] Area excursion is also reduced. At echocardiography, significant tricuspid annular dilation is defined by a diastolic diameter of greater than 21 mm/m² (>35 mm).[10] In vitro bench tests have shown that a 40% annulus dilation is enough to cause significant TR.[24] At CT, increased septolateral diameter of 41.2 mm ± 5.6 mm and area of 16.1 cm² ± 2.9 cm², up to 18.5 cm² ± 6.9 cm² in diastole were observed in patients with TR greater than or equal to 3+.[12,17] Annulus calcification is infrequent in the setting of fTR.

In a minority of cases, fTR can be caused by isolated annulus dilation[20,25] due to RA dilation as primum movens, without significant right ventricular remodeling and leaflet tethering, at least in the early stages. This atrial fTR mostly occurs in the setting of long-standing atrial fibrillation. This form is usually more benign, having in itself no associated left-sided heart disease, pulmonary hypertension (PH), or RV dysfunction (until late evolution to RV volume overload). According to its pathophysiologic mechanism, it responds well to tricuspid annuloplasty repair.

Most frequently, fTR is caused by right ventricular pressure/volume overload, leading to ventricular remodeling with both tricuspid annular dilation and leaflet tethering. In this

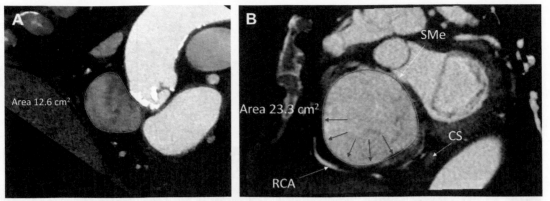

Fig. 3. CT scan en face measurement of the tricuspid valve orifice in diastole in a healthy subject (*A*) compared with a patient affected by severe fTR (*B*). CS, coronary sinus; SMe, septum membranosum. Red arrows depict annulus dilatation.

kind of ventricular fTR, the most common cause of RV overload is PH due to present or past left-sided heart disease. Less commonly, primitive PH (pressure overload) or congenital heart defects (volume overload) are responsible.[26]

Fig. 5 depicts exemplified the progressive stages of ventricular fTR:

- At an early-phase, annular dilation develops. Both RA and RV dilation can be seen but without significant RV dysfunction or leaflet tethering and TR can be mild to severe depending on the severity of annular enlargement and residual coaptation length of the leaflets.

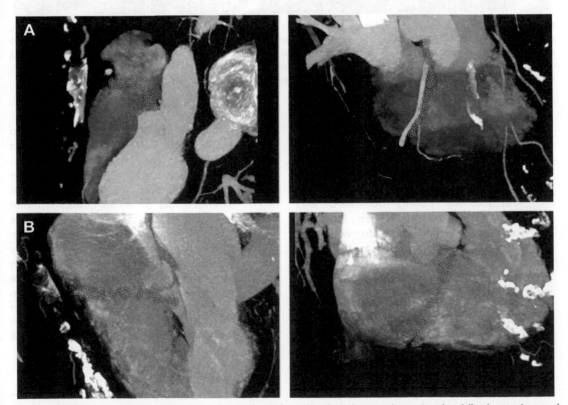

Fig. 4. CT scan 3-D reconstruction of the tricuspid annulus. The physiologic tridimensional saddle shape observed in a healthy subject (*A*) is lost in a patient affected by severe TR (*B*), with annulus dilation and flattening. On left panels: left-cranial-oblique projections. On right panels: right-oblique projections.

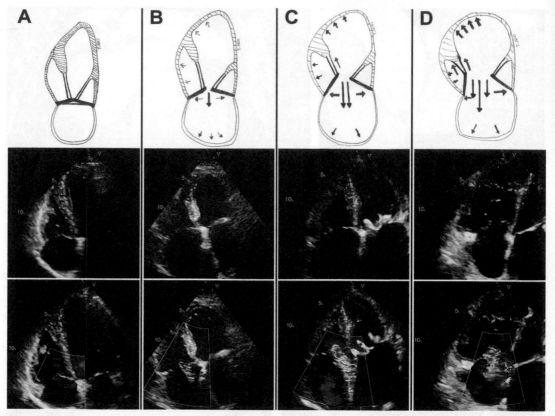

Fig. 5. Schematic and echocardiographic representation of progressive stages of fTR. Normal valve, no RA or RV dilation, and no significant TR (*A*); annulus dilation, no significant tethering, mild RV dilation, and variable degrees of TR from mild to severe can be observed at this stage (*B*); annulus dilation and leaflet tethering, dilated RV, and severe TR (*C*); and annulus dilation, severe tethering with complete loss of coaptation, severe RV remodeling, and massive TR (*D*). Top row: schematic illustration; Middle row: echocardiographic anatomical detail; Bottom row: echocardiographic TR at color-doppler.

This stage is easily repairable with an annuloplasty technique.

- At a later time, with ongoing remodeling, the dilated RV creates tethering forces due to free wall and papillary muscles displacement pulling downward and outward the tricuspid leaflets, impairing coaptation and leading to worsening degrees of fTR.[27] Similar to the mitral AV valve on the left side, excessive tricuspid leaflet tethering is a known predictor of TR recurrence after surgical annuloplasty. Tethering distance 8 mm to 10 mm, tented area greater than 1.6 cm^2, and tented volume greater than or equal to 2.3 mL were all found associated with worse follow-up TR degrees.[28–30] Given these findings, annuloplasty alone should be considered with caution in the presence of severe leaflet tethering. Some leaflet repair technique (such as the clover[31] or the leaflet augmentation[32]) can be added to annuloplasty to improve the efficacy and durability of repair in this setting.

- As the RV continues to deteriorate, leaflet tethering further worsens, leading to extended loss of leaflet coaptation that can result in more than severe TR degrees (so-called massive TR and torrential TR). At this stage, the RV is usually severely dilated, spherical, and dysfunctioning. In such a scenario any repair attempt is futile and replacement, if any, should be considered based on residual RV function and pulmonary vascular resistance, which are the 2 final criteria to decide about tricuspid intervention.

Right Ventricle Function

RV remodeling is the underlying primary pathologic mechanism of most cases of fTR; therefore, the assessment of RV function is fundamental at every stage of the disease. In most cases it still relies mostly on echo, but, as discussed previously, its evaluation remains challenging. Accepted echocardiographic cutoff values for nonsignificant right-sided chamber enlargement obtained from the echocardiographic apical 4-chamber view are mid-RV dimension less than or equal to 33 mm, RV end-diastolic area less than or equal to 28 cm^2, RV end-systolic area less than or equal to 16 cm^2, and RV fractional area change greater than 32%.[10] In clinical practice, TAPSE less than 15 mm, tricuspid annulus systolic velocity less than 11 cm/s, and RV end-systolic area greater than 20 cm^2 can be used to identify patients with RV dysfunction.[33] Both the TAPSE and the systolic velocity, however, are less accurate in patients with severe TR, and parameters that are less load-dependent (ie, longitudinal strain and strain rate) could be more useful in this setting.

Unfortunately, many patients are currently referred late for fTR intervention, when RV remodeling is too advanced and irreversible. At this stage the patients are at extreme risk for conventional surgery and are left untreated.

In such a scenario, dobutamine stress echocardiography and an intensive therapy regimen with intravenous diuretics and inotropes to optimize the RV may be helpful in patient selection.

Pulmonary Hypertension and Vascular Resistance

PH is frequently associated with significant TR; it is one of the causes of fTR and one of the factors associated with impaired outcomes after treatment of TR.[34] Regarding operative decision making, PH and its relationship with RV function must be carefully studied. Specifically, in a patient with a long history of heart disease, irreversibly increased pulmonary vascular resistance must be ruled out with right heart catheterization. Moreover, it should be remembered that low pulmonary pressures in a known advanced stage of disease with previous PH may suggest severe end-stage RV dysfunction. Also, it should be remembered that the estimation of pulmonary pressures by echocardiography and of cardiac output by invasive thermodilution method may be unreliable in the setting of severe TR.

Timing of Intervention

From a clinical perspective, 3 main kinds of fTR patients can be distinguished today.

The first consists of patients with concomitant left-sided valvular heart disease. A vast majority of all tricuspid interventions are currently performed in association with other (most frequently mitral) procedures.[35] In such patients

there is a clear indication to correction of fTR at the time of left-sided operation in TR if severe (European Guidelines class of recommendation I, level of evidence C).[26] In cases of less than severe fTR, however, opportunity of intervention is debated, and there are conflicting data regarding the evolution of TR during follow-up. Some recent evidence suggests that a nondilated tricuspid annulus and an effectively repaired degenerative mitral valve disease may be associated with a low rate of TR progression during follow-up.[36–38] According to current guidelines, surgery should be considered in patients with mild or moderate secondary TR with a dilated annulus (≥40 mm or >21 mm/m^2) undergoing left-sided valve surgery (class IIa C).

A second group is formed by patients with isolated atrial annular dilation. As discussed previously, this is a rare, low-risk, easily repairable anatomical setting. Although not specifically addressed in the current guidelines, such patients should be operated on before the onset of severe RV dysfunction or severe pulmonary vascular disease.

The third is patients affected by isolated fTR after left-sided heart surgery. These are usually the sickest patients, operated on several years before, with long-lasting RV overload and several comorbidities.[39] Given their advanced stage, valve replacement is usually required in these patients. Some of them also have a rheumatic component that makes their valves even more likely to require replacement. After left-sided valve surgery, surgery should be considered in patients with severe TR who are symptomatic or have progressive RV enlargement/dysfunction, in the absence of left-sided valve dysfunction, severe right or left ventricular dysfunction, and severe pulmonary vascular disease (class IIa C).

For decades a vicious circle of late referral–poor outcomes has been and continues to be perpetuated, with the tricuspid valve largely neglected and becoming the now famous "forgotten valve." Indeed, historically TR has been thought to "improve or disappear after mitral replacement" and, therefore, it was believed that "tricuspid replacement is seldom necessary."[40] Also TR is per se asymptomatic for a long period of time, and, due to its high pendence from loading conditions, it usually responds well to diuretic therapy until advanced stages of the disease. Patients were rarely submitted to tricuspid surgery, mostly when markedly symptomatic in an advanced stage of the disease. Not surprisingly, early surgical mortality was very high (up to 35% for tricuspid redo operations[41]), which in turn further discouraged the cardiology community from referring patients affected by TR for earlier surgery.

Over past few years, technical improvements (like performing beating heart tricuspid surgery), refined patient selection, and overall improved knowledge derived from surgery have led to better outcomes after tricuspid valve procedures (8% overall acute mortality after tricuspid surgery).[35] Nevertheless, many patients continue to be referred late to treatment. Even today these patients, if treated, are characterized by elevated procedural risk, difficult advanced anatomies (often requiring replacement), and impaired outcomes.

More than the mere restoration of valve function, RV unloading is the early target and RV reverse remodeling is the long-term goal of any TR intervention. To achieve these objectives earlier treatment, patient selection and technical performance (safety and efficacy) are all fundamental.

IMPLICATIONS FOR PERCUTANEOUS THERAPIES

The spread of percutaneous transcatheter technologies has finally reached the tricuspid valve.[3] Several important implications for these devices can be derived from tricuspid anatomy, pathophysiology, and surgical experience:

- Tricuspid anatomy is huge. It is the biggest of the heart valves, bigger than the mitral, and it gets even bigger in the setting of severe TR. The issue is clear if the mean CT-measured area of a regurgitant tricuspid valve is compared with the cross-sectional area of an aortic 29-mm SAPIEN 3 (Edwards Lifescience, Irvine, California) valve: approximately 17 cm^2 versus 6.8 cm^2 respectively. Dedicated prostheses sizes and shapes will be required to address such big anatomy. On the other hand, the significant distance between the tricuspid valve and the RV outflow tract means that RV outflow tract obstruction after transcatheter valve replacement will be rare.
- Tricuspid leaflet and annular tissues are more fragile than those of the mitral valve. Therefore, careful engagement and manipulation with catheters, anchors, and devices must be conducted.
- Tricuspid anatomy is complex and rarely calcific. Differently from the aortic and similar to the mitral, purposely developed fixation mechanisms will be required. On the other hand, differently from the mitral valve, the low pressures

in the right side of the heart could make easier and more durable device fixation into soft tissue.
- Several important structures lie in close proximity to the tricuspid annulus, the most important being the conduction system (both AV node and His bundle), the AV septum, the ostium of the coronary sinus, and the RCA. These may be directly damaged during device implantation but also distorted after the device is activated. Specifically, perforation/kinking/impingement of RCA, which is rare but can happen during surgery,[42] may happen with several transcatheter devices targeting the annulus.[43–45] The fact that RCA is closer to the tricuspid annulus at the level of the posterior annulus rather than the anterior annulus should guide patient selection and procedure execution.
- Given the complex soft tissue valve anatomy, its high variability, and the numerous delicate surrounding structures, careful preprocedural planning with 3-D echo and CT reconstructions is fundamental to tailor the treatment to the specific patient, maximizing safety and efficacy. Useful specific landmarks can be identified with CT scan, such as the septum membranosum for the anteroseptal commissure with His bundle and the ostium of the coronary sinus for the AV node on one side and the posteroseptal commissure on the other.
- As per the tricuspid anatomy and anterior position in the heart (far from the esophagus with several other structures between them), intraprocedural echocardiographic imaging guidance is more challenging that in the mitral valve, especially for the anterior tricuspid leaflet. The leaflets are more difficult to see and leaflet grasping more difficult to appreciate. Shadowing caused by mitral and aortic prostheses can significantly impair tricuspid visualization. 3-D and intracardiac echocardiography can be useful tools to improve the intraprocedural imaging.[46]
- Annulus enlargement is a major mechanism of fTR in almost every fTR case. Patients with isolated annulus enlargement represent ideal candidates for annuloplasty repair devices.
- Leaflet tethering predicts failure of surgical annuloplasty. Patients with

concomitant or prevalent leaflet tethering should be considered for a combined leaflet procedure (edge-to-edge, spacer) or replacement.

- Transcatheter technologies do not carry the heavy trauma of surgery but severe RV dysfunction and severe pulmonary vascular resistance, which are the real absolute contraindications to TR correction, remain fearsome caveats for any intervention that significantly reduces TR, independently from its access route. The subsequent afterload mismatch, as already seen in the mitral setting,[47] can cause RV failure.
- Thanks to their true minimally invasiveness, with no need of open-chest open-heart approach, transcatheter technologies could
  - Treat inoperable/high-risk patients who currently have no options
  - Allow earlier intervention
  - Allow both concomitant and multiple and staged procedures in patients with multiple valvular heart disease, with lower risk compared with surgery
  - Allow unconventional anatomic procedures in the setting of difficult anatomies, such as spacer devices (to unload the RV), and extra-anatomic prostheses implantation (to relief peripheral venous congestion)
- Given the multifaceted patients profile and complex intraprocedural anatomy, a multidisciplinary heart team approach is recommended to deal with the spectrum of TR pathology.

SUMMARY

The tricuspid valve presents complex anatomy and function, with many nearby structures that require careful consideration. The RV plays a crucial role in fTR, although its assessment remains to be fully clarified. Understanding the anatomy and the function of the tricuspid AV valve within the right heart is fundamental for the development of transcatheter tricuspid valve technologies. Careful preprocedural planning with 3-D echo and CT is crucial to tailor the treatment to specific patients and reach optimal safety and efficacy.

ACKNOWLEDGMENTS

The authors would like to thank Dr Teodora Nisi for the hand drawings.

REFERENCES

1. Mack MJ, Leon MB, Smith CR, et al. 5-year outcomes of transcatheter aortic valve replacement or surgical aortic valve replacement for high surgical risk patients with aortic stenosis (PARTNER 1): a randomised controlled trial. Lancet 2015;385(9986): 2477–84.
2. Feldman T, Kar S, Elmariah S, et al. Randomized comparison of percutaneous repair and surgery for mitral regurgitation: 5-year results of EVEREST II. J Am Coll Cardiol 2015;66(25):2844–54.
3. Rodes-Cabau J, Hahn RT, Latib A, et al. Transcatheter therapies for treating tricuspid regurgitation. J Am Coll Cardiol 2016;67(15):1829–45.
4. Naoum C, Blanke P, Cavalcante JL, et al. Cardiac computed tomography and magnetic resonance imaging in the evaluation of mitral and tricuspid valve disease: implications for transcatheter interventions. Circ Cardiovasc Imaging 2017;10(3) [pii: e005331].
5. Saremi F, Hassani C, Millan-Nunez V, et al. Imaging evaluation of tricuspid valve: analysis of morphology and function with CT and MRI. AJR Am J Roentgenol 2015;204(5):W531–42.
6. Westaby S, Karp RB, Blackstone EH, et al. Adult human valve dimensions and their surgical significance. Am J Cardiol 1984;53(4):552–6.
7. Kwan J, Kim GC, Jeon MJ, et al. 3D geometry of a normal tricuspid annulus during systole: a comparison study with the mitral annulus using real-time 3D echocardiography. Eur J Echocardiogr 2007; 8(5):375–83.
8. Fukuda S, Saracino G, Matsumura Y, et al. Three-dimensional geometry of the tricuspid annulus in healthy subjects and in patients with functional tricuspid regurgitation: a real-time, 3-dimensional echocardiographic study. Circulation 2006; 114(1 Suppl):I492–8.
9. Rudski LG, Lai WW, Afilalo J, et al. Guidelines for the echocardiographic assessment of the right heart in adults: a report from the American Society of Echocardiography endorsed by the European Association of Echocardiography, a registered branch of the European Society of Cardiology, and the Canadian Society of Echocardiography. J Am Soc Echocardiogr 2010;23(7):685–713 [quiz: 786–8].
10. Lancellotti P, Tribouilloy C, Hagendorff A, et al. Recommendations for the echocardiographic assessment of native valvular regurgitation: an executive summary from the European Association of Cardiovascular Imaging. Eur Heart J Cardiovasc Imaging 2013;14(7):611–44.
11. Hahn RT. State-of-the-art review of echocardiographic imaging in the evaluation and treatment of functional tricuspid regurgitation. Circ Cardiovasc Imaging 2016;9(12) [pii:e005332].

12. Hinzpeter R, Eberhard M, Burghard P, et al. Computed tomography in patients with tricuspid regurgitation prior to transcatheter valve repair: dynamic analysis of the annulus with an individually tailored contrast media protocol. EuroIntervention 2017;12(15):e1828–36.

13. Silver MD, Lam JH, Ranganathan N, et al. Morphology of the human tricuspid valve. Circulation 1971;43(3):333–48.

14. James TN. Morphology of the human atrioventricular node, with remarks pertinent to its electrophysiology. Am Heart J 1961;62:756–71.

15. Titus JL. Normal anatomy of the human cardiac conduction system. Mayo Clin Proc 1973;48(1):24–30.

16. Ueda A, McCarthy KP, Sanchez-Quintana D, et al. Right atrial appendage and vestibule: further anatomical insights with implications for invasive electrophysiology. Europace 2013;15(5):728–34.

17. van Rosendael PJ, Kamperidis V, Kong WK, et al. Computed tomography for planning transcatheter tricuspid valve therapy. Eur Heart J 2017;38(9):665–74.

18. Nath J, Foster E, Heidenreich PA. Impact of tricuspid regurgitation on long-term survival. J Am Coll Cardiol 2004;43(3):405–9.

19. Trichon BH, O'Connor CM. Secondary mitral and tricuspid regurgitation accompanying left ventricular systolic dysfunction: is it important, and how is it treated? Am Heart J 2002;144(3):373–6.

20. Mutlak D, Lessick J, Reisner SA, et al. Echocardiography-based spectrum of severe tricuspid regurgitation: the frequency of apparently idiopathic tricuspid regurgitation. J Am Soc Echocardiogr 2007;20(4):405–8.

21. Topilsky Y, Tribouilloy C, Michelena HI, et al. Pathophysiology of tricuspid regurgitation: quantitative Doppler echocardiographic assessment of respiratory dependence. Circulation 2010;122(15):1505–13.

22. Badano LP, Muraru D, Enriquez-Sarano M. Assessment of functional tricuspid regurgitation. Eur Heart J 2013;34(25):1875–85.

23. Badano LP, Agricola E, Perez de Isla L, et al. Evaluation of the tricuspid valve morphology and function by transthoracic real-time three-dimensional echocardiography. Eur J Echocardiogr 2009;10(4):477–84.

24. Spinner EM, Shannon P, Buice D, et al. In vitro characterization of the mechanisms responsible for functional tricuspid regurgitation. Circulation 2011;124(8):920–9.

25. Girard SE, Nishimura RA, Warnes CA, et al. Idiopathic annular dilation: a rare cause of isolated severe tricuspid regurgitation. J Heart Valve Dis 2000;9(2):283–7.

26. Vahanian A, Alfieri O, Andreotti F, et al. Guidelines on the management of valvular heart disease (version 2012): the Joint Task Force on the Management of Valvular Heart Disease of the European Society of Cardiology (ESC) and the European Association for Cardio-Thoracic Surgery (EACTS). Eur J Cardiothorac Surg 2012;42(4):S1–44.

27. Kim HK, Kim YJ, Park JS, et al. Determinants of the severity of functional tricuspid regurgitation. Am J Cardiol 2006;98(2):236–42.

28. Fukuda S, Gillinov AM, McCarthy PM, et al. Determinants of recurrent or residual functional tricuspid regurgitation after tricuspid annuloplasty. Circulation 2006;114(1 Suppl):I582–7.

29. Min SY, Song JM, Kim JH, et al. Geometric changes after tricuspid annuloplasty and predictors of residual tricuspid regurgitation: a real-time three-dimensional echocardiography study. Eur Heart J 2010;31(23):2871–80.

30. Fukuda S, Gillinov AM, McCarthy PM, et al. Echocardiographic follow-up of tricuspid annuloplasty with a new three-dimensional ring in patients with functional tricuspid regurgitation. J Am Soc Echocardiogr 2007;20(11):1236–42.

31. De Bonis M, Lapenna E, Di Sanzo S, et al. Long-term results (up to 14 years) of the clover technique for the treatment of complex tricuspid valve regurgitationdagger. Eur J Cardiothorac Surg 2017;52(1):125–30.

32. Dreyfus GD, Raja SG, John Chan KM. Tricuspid leaflet augmentation to address severe tethering in functional tricuspid regurgitation. Eur J Cardiothorac Surg 2008;34(4):908–10.

33. Haddad F, Doyle R, Murphy DJ, et al. Right ventricular function in cardiovascular disease, part II: pathophysiology, clinical importance, and management of right ventricular failure. Circulation 2008;117(13):1717–31.

34. Mutlak D, Aronson D, Lessick J, et al. Functional tricuspid regurgitation in patients with pulmonary hypertension: is pulmonary artery pressure the only determinant of regurgitation severity? Chest 2009;135(1):115–21.

35. Kilic A, Saha-Chaudhuri P, Rankin JS, et al. Trends and outcomes of tricuspid valve surgery in North America: an analysis of more than 50,000 patients from the Society of Thoracic Surgeons database. Ann Thorac Surg 2013;96(5):1546–52 [discussion: 1552].

36. David TE, David CM, Fan CS, et al. Tricuspid regurgitation is uncommon after mitral valve repair for degenerative diseases. J Thorac Cardiovasc Surg 2017;154(1):110–22.e1.

37. Sordelli C, Lancellotti P, Carlomagno G, et al. Tricuspid annular size and regurgitation progression after surgical repair for degenerative mitral regurgitation. Am J Cardiol 2016;118(3):424–31.

38. Dreyfus GD, Corbi PJ, Chan KM, et al. Secondary tricuspid regurgitation or dilatation: which should

be the criteria for surgical repair? Ann Thorac Surg 2005;79(1):127–32.

39. Buzzatti N, Iaci G, Taramasso M, et al. Long-term outcomes of tricuspid valve replacement after previous left-side heart surgery. Eur J Cardiothorac Surg 2014;46(4):713–9 [discussion: 719].

40. Braunwald NS, Ross J Jr, Morrow AG. Conservative management of tricuspid regurgitation in patients undergoing mitral valve replacement. Circulation 1967;35(4 Suppl):I63–9.

41. Bernal JM, Morales D, Revuelta C, et al. Reoperations after tricuspid valve repair. J Thorac Cardiovasc Surg 2005;130(2):498–503.

42. Diez-Villanueva P, Gutierrez-Ibanes E, Cuerpo-Caballero GP, et al. Direct injury to right coronary artery in patients undergoing tricuspid annuloplasty. Ann Thorac Surg 2014;97(4):1300–5.

43. Latib A, Agricola E, Pozzoli A, et al. First-in-man implantation of a tricuspid annular remodeling device for functional tricuspid regurgitation. JACC Cardiovasc Interv 2015;8(13):e211–214.

44. Schofer J, Bijuklic K, Tiburtius C, et al. First-in-human transcatheter tricuspid valve repair in a patient with severely regurgitant tricuspid valve. J Am Coll Cardiol 2015;65(12):1190–5.

45. Kuwata S, Taramasso M, Nietlispach F, et al. Transcatheter tricuspid valve repair toward a surgical standard: first-in-man report of direct annuloplasty with a cardioband device to treat severe functional tricuspid regurgitation. Eur Heart J 2017;38(16):1261.

46. Ancona F, Stella S, Taramasso M, et al. Multimodality imaging of the tricuspid valve with implication for percutaneous repair approaches. Heart 2017; 103(14):1073–81.

47. Melisurgo G, Ajello S, Pappalardo F, et al. Afterload mismatch after MitraClip insertion for functional mitral regurgitation. Am J Cardiol 2014; 113(11):1844–50.

Interventional Imaging of the Tricuspid Valve

Francesco Ancona, MD[a], Eustachio Agricola, MD[a],*, Stefano Stella, MD[a], Cristina Capogrosso, MD[a], Claudia Marini, MD[a], Alberto Margonato, MD[a], Rebecca T. Hahn, MD[b]

KEYWORDS

- Tricuspid regurgitation • Imaging • Interventional echocardiography
- Percutaneous tricuspid valve intervention • Transcatheter tricuspid valve repair/replacement

KEY POINTS

- Transcatheter tricuspid valve interventions (TTVIs) are emerging as attractive alternative options for patients affected by functional tricuspid regurgitation (FTR) due to some degree of annular dilation and leaflet tethering.
- Because of the complex nature of the tricuspid valve (TV), a comprehensive assessment should be performed from multiple transthoracic and transesophageal windows, including a 3-dimensional evaluation.
- The procedural planning for TTVIs is based on a multimodality imaging approach (based on echocardiography and computed tomography scan), aiming to define FTR, TV morphology, and anatomic relationships.
- A good target for TTVIs seems to be FTR with predominant annular dilatation and modest apical remodeling, without severe dysfunction of the right ventricle and/or severe pulmonary hypertension.
- Intraprocedural guidance is based mainly on transesophageal echocardiography (seldom transthoracic) and fluoroscopy, with the recent introduction of fusion imaging.

INTRODUCTION

Functional tricuspid regurgitation (FTR) impacts negatively on the prognosis of patients with mitral valve disease and advanced left ventricular dysfunction.[1] Usually these patients are managed conservatively[2] until advanced stages of disease when the surgical option becomes prohibitive.[3] Therefore, reasonable low-risk, less-invasive transcatheter tricuspid valve interventions (TTVIs) are emerging as attractive alternative options.

However, the dimensions and the angulation of the tricuspid annulus (TA) in relation to the caval veins, the slow flow and trabeculated structure of the right-heart, and the lack of annular calcification make the percutaneous implantation of a bioprosthesis challenging[4] and, thus, was performed only as valve-in-valve or valve-in-ring procedures.[5,6] The following percutaneous options are under development:

1. Implantation of a bioprosthetic valve in both caval veins[7]

Disclosure Statement: Dr E. Agricola has served as a consultant for Edwards, Valtech, Abbott, and 4Tech. R.T. Hahn is the National principal investigator for the SCOUT trial for which she receives no compensation. She is the Echo Core Lab Director for several tricuspid device trials for which she receives no compensation. She is a consultant for Abbott Structural.
[a] Echocardiography Laboratory, Clinical Cardiology Unit, San Raffaele Scientific Institute, Via Olgettina 60, Milano 20132, Italy; [b] Columbia University Medical Center, New York Presbyterian Hospital, 177 Fort Washington Avenue, New York, NY 10032, USA
* Corresponding author.
E-mail address: agricola.eustachio@hsr.it

Intervent Cardiol Clin 7 (2018) 13–29
https://doi.org/10.1016/j.iccl.2017.08.010

2. Percutaneous tricuspid valve (TV) repair mimicking the surgical Kay procedure (TriCinch System, 4Tech Cardio Ltd, Galway, Ireland; Trialign System, Mitralign, Inc, Boston, MA)[8–10]
3. Percutaneous TV repair targeting leaflets (MitraClip System, Abbott Vascular, Abbott Park, IL)[11]
4. Direct percutaneous TV annuloplasty (Cardioband, Edwards Lifesciences, Irvine, CA)[12]
5. Transcatheter delivery of a spacer providing a surface for leaflet coaptation (FORMA Spacer, Edwards Lifesciences, Irvine, CA)[13]
6. TV replacement[14]

As for other transcatheter procedures, pre-procedural planning and intraprocedural monitoring are fundamental. All potential candidates should be screened with transthoracic echocardiography (TTE) and, if eligibility seems plausible, a second-level imaging evaluation with transesophageal echocardiography (TEE); in some cases, a computed tomography (CT) scan is mandatory in order to evaluate all the anatomic details needed. The screening process is also aimed at tailoring the procedure and choosing the best option for every single patient.

The intraprocedural imaging, mainly by TEE and sometimes TTE, is essential to monitor all the procedural steps, to check the results, and to timely detect complications.

TRICUSPID VALVE ANATOMY
Normal Anatomy
The right atrioventricular valve is the largest and most inferiorly positioned valve; its functional anatomy can be divided into 4 components: the fibrous annulus, the leaflets, the papillary muscles, and the chordal attachments.[15,16] The anatomic position of the tricuspid annular plane is nearly vertical and approximately 45° from the sagittal plane. The annulus is triangular or ovoid as well as saddle shaped superiorly (atrially), displaced in the anteroseptal portion near the right ventricular (RV) outflow tract and aortic valve and the posterolateral portion, and inferiorly (apically) displaced in the postero-septal portion near the inflow of the coronary sinus and the anterolateral segment.[17] Unlike the mitral valve, there is no fibrous continuity with the corresponding semilunar valve. Like the mitral valve, annular dynamism contributes to leaflet closure.[15,17–19] Normal tricuspid annular circumference and area in healthy subjects are 12 ± 1 cm and 11 ± 2 cm^2, respectively.[17,20]

During atrial systole and again in late ventricular systole/early diastole, there is a significant increase in annular area ($29.6\% \pm 5.5\%$) as well as circumference. Importantly, the right coronary artery courses within the right coronary sulcus and is typically embedded in fat, approximately 5 to 8 mm above the right fibrous annulus.[21] This relationship can vary, however, and should be understood before surgical or transcatheter-based therapy.

There is significant variability in the number of TV leaflets, with reports between 2 and 6 leaflets.[22] The increased number is most commonly due to the presence of supernumerary and/or commissural cusps: most cases in one pathologic study had 4 leaflets with the location of the fourth between the anterior and posterior leaflets. The most common description of the tricuspid, nonetheless, is of a 3-leaflet valve with leaflets varying in both circumferential (annular) and radial size. Because of the vertical position of the tricuspid annulus, the appropriate anatomic names of the leaflets are *antero-superior*, *septal*, and *inferior*. However, the nomenclature commonly used for these leaflets are *anterior*, *septal*, and *posterior*. The anterior leaflet is the longest radial leaflet with the largest area and the greatest motion. The septal leaflet is the shortest in the radial direction and the least mobile. This short septal leaflet is attached to the TA directly above the interventricular septum with several third-order chordae attached directly to the septum; it is inserted into the septum 10 mm or less apical to the septal insertion of the anterior mitral leaflet (ie, apically displaced). The posterior (or mural or inferior) leaflet may have multiple scallops and is the shortest circumferentially; however, it may not be clearly separated from the anterior leaflet in approximately 10% of patients. Anatomic landmarks for each leaflet vary significantly depending on the size and shape of the annulus; however, the commissure between the septal and posterior leaflets (which are always clearly separated) is usually located near the entrance of the coronary sinus to the right atrium. A normal TV area is between 7 and 9 cm^2 and is, thus, the largest of the 4 cardiac valves. Because of its large size and the low-pressure differences between the right atrium and ventricle, peak transtricuspid diastolic velocities are typically lower than 1 m/s with mean gradients less than 2 mm Hg.

The papillary muscles of the TV also exhibit significant variability.[23,24] The large anterior papillary muscle is the most consistent, arising from the anterior wall near the trabeculations, which incorporate the moderator band. The papillary muscle typically has a single head and less commonly 2 heads and primarily supports the anterior leaflet but also the commissure between the anterior and posterior leaflets. The small medial papillary muscle arises from the posterior septal band and supports the septal and anterior leaflets. The posterior papillary muscle, on the other hand, most frequently has 2 heads but can have up to 4. It supports the commissure between the posterior and septal leaflets. Numerous direct chordal attachments to the ventricular wall with no septal papillary muscle can be seen in 21% to 93% of patients. Otherwise 1 septal papillary muscle head is more common than 2 heads. Chordal attachments are also different for each leaflet: the septal leaflet has the most chordal attachments; rough zone chordae are the primary support for the anterior leaflet, and basal chordae are seen attached to the inferior leaflet.

Other important anatomies for interventions include the orifices of the venae cavae and coronary sinus.[21] The superior vena cava (SVC) is superiorly positioned, behind the right atrial appendage and directly adjacent to the interatrial septum. The inferior vena caval orifice is very large, and the anterosuperior horn of its eustachian valve (the tendon of Todaro) forms the posterior border of the triangle of Koch and is used to help identify the position of the atrioventricular node. The third vascular entrance into the right atrium is the coronary sinus. This orifice of the coronary sinus is along the medial wall of the right atrium, approximately 2 cm behind the body of the septal cusp, most commonly at the commissure between the septal and posterior leaflet. This orifice should be distinguished from the inferomedial recess of the atrium, a blind pouch lateral to the coronary sinus. Along with the tendon of Todaro, the Thebesius valve of the coronary sinus forms the inferior border; the anterior-septal leaflet commissure forms the superior border of the triangle of Koch.

Tricuspid Anatomy with Functional Tricuspid Regurgitation

When functional dilatation occurs, the septal portion of the annulus that is supported by attachment to the muscular septum is typically spared, and so the annulus primarily dilates along the anterior and posterior leaflet attachments, causing the annulus to become more circular and planar.[18] Greater degrees of TR are associated with larger annular areas, larger right and left atrial volumes, a more circular annular

shape, and RV dilatation.[25] Animal models of TR have suggested that greater degrees of TR are associated with greater "stretch" of the posterior leaflet (as compared with the anterior or septal leaflets) with greater annular dilatation or RV dilatation and/or with displacement of the papillary muscles, with little effect from the loss of the annulus' saddle-shape.[26] Recent studies, however, have also shown that significant anatomic differences in RV, valve, and annular anatomy may occur based on the cause of functional TR. With idiopathic TR, there was marked basal RV dilatation associated with annular dilatation in the absence of leaflet tethering, with relatively normal RV length (RV conical deformation). With functional TR associated with pulmonary hypertension there was significant lengthening of the RV with less basal dilatation (and low basal/midventricular diameter ratios) but more midventricular dilatation, resulting in both increased tenting as well as elliptical/spherical RV deformation.[27] Numerous authors have also explored the relationship between tenting of the leaflets and severity of TR with tenting areas and volumes correlating with TR severity and with recurrence and outcomes following surgical repair.[28,29] These differences of RV and tricuspid annular anatomy may also have significant impact on the success of different transcatheter approaches.

ECHOCARDIOGRAPHIC IMAGING OF THE TRICUSPID VALVE

Recent guidelines from the American Society of Echocardiography (ASE)[5] outline the recommended TTE views for performing a comprehensive evaluation of the valve[30] and measurement of the right heart chamber.[31] New ASE guidelines for performing a comprehensive TEE also emphasize imaging of the TV.[32] Finally, the approach to 3-dimensional (3D) imaging of the TV has been addressed in both guidelines[33] and reviews.

Transthoracic Echocardiography
Because of the complex nature of the TV and the difficulty in visualizing all 3 leaflets in a single 2-dimensional (2D) plane, a comprehensive assessment of the TV should be performed from multiple transthoracic windows. Recent ASE guidelines outline the recommended views for performing a comprehensive evaluation of the RV and TV; however, identification of the tricuspid leaflets from standard transthoracic views remains controversial, in part because of the variability of imaging planes that can be

acquired from varying degrees of transducer angulation as well as the significant anatomic variability described earlier.[19,34] Understanding the anatomy of the TV and adjacent structures should help clarify the imaging planes and allow for a more accurate identification of the tricuspid leaflets.

A few anatomic caveats are important. First, the commissure between the anterior and septal leaflet is adjacent to the noncoronary cusp of the aortic valve; the right coronary cusp is adjacent to only the anterior leaflet. Second, although a small (anterior) portion of the septal leaflet may be seen if the aorta is in view, most of the septal leaflet is attached to the interventricular septum. Third, the coronary sinus enters the right atrium at the commissure between the septal and posterior leaflet. Finally, the right atrial appendage is directly superior to the anterior leaflet. Any 2-chamber imaging plane of the RV (parasternal inflow or apical 2-chamber views) will tend to image the anterior and posterior leaflets as long as the anterior (curved, right atrial appendage in view) and posterior (flat, on the diaphragm) walls of the RV are imaged.[35] A 4-chamber view, on the other hand, will frequently image the septal and posterior leaflet, although slight anterior angulation (with or without aorta in view) will image septal and anterior leaflets and slight posterior angulation (with or without the coronary sinus in view) will image the septal and posterior leaflets. From the parasternal short-axis views, an extreme anterior angulation may result in imaging of a single large anterior leaflet or the anterior and posterior leaflet.[19,34,36]

Imaging of the right heart is similarly nuanced because of the unusual shape of the RV, discontinuity of the atrioventricular valve and outflow tract, and position in the chest. The recent ASE chamber quantification guideline[31] recommends 3 apical 4-chamber views for imaging the RV: apical 4 chamber, RV-focused apical 4 chamber, and modified apical 4 chamber. Although the RV has typically been measured from the standard apical 4-chamber view, the new guidelines suggest measuring the RV from the dedicated view focused on the RV because the entire RV free wall is imaged. Other measurements of RV size and function are extensively reviewed in the ASE's guidelines.[31] RV wall thickness is measured from subcostal views, which may also allow Doppler alignments of the tricuspid regurgitation (TR) jet. In addition, an assessment of right atrial filling pressure should be made from the evaluation of size and respirophasic variability of the inferior vena cava (IVC).

Transesophageal Echocardiography

The ASE's current guidelines for performing a comprehensive TEE examination[32] include additional images, many of which are intended to improve imaging of the TV. In addition, the TEE examination of the TV should include imaging from several depths and multiplane angles. Given the position of the heart in relation to the esophagus and stomach, midesophageal, distal esophageal, shallow transgastric, as well as deep transgastric views may bring the probe close to the TV for both 2D and 3D imaging. Many imaging planes may be similar to TTE imaging, and the same imaging caveats are worth noting.

Multilevel imaging begins at the midesophageal depth. The 4-chamber view permits visualization of the septal and, typically, the anterior leaflet; simultaneous biplane imaging may help clarify which leaflet is imaged particularly given the high variability of the number and relative size of each leaflet. Rotating from the 4-chamber view at 0° to a midesophageal inflow-outflow view at 90° images the anterior leaflet (adjacent to the aorta) and the opposing posterior leaflet. Because the lower right heart border is close to the diaphragm, slow insertion brings the TEE probe to the distal esophagus just proximal to the gastroesophageal junction; from this imaging plane, there may not be a left atrium in view, only the right atrium and coronary sinus. Because this view of the TV is unobstructed by left heart structures, it is ideal for performing a comprehensive evaluation of TV function and for acquiring 3D volumes of the TV. At 0° from this level, the posterior leaflet, which sits on the diaphragm, is typically seen particularly if the coronary sinus is in view. The opposing anterior leaflet can be identified adjacent to the right atrial appendage. Advancing the TEE probe into the stomach results in transgastric views. At 0°, right and anteflexion will result in the inflow-outflow view again with imaging of the anterior (adjacent to the aorta) and posterior (adjacent to the diaphragm) leaflets. Rotating the multiangle probe 60° to 90° results in the only 2D view that provides simultaneous visualization of all 3 TV leaflets with the posterior leaflet in the near field, the anterior leaflet in far field, and the septal leaflet adjacent to the septum. Advancing the TEE probe further into the stomach along with rightward anterior flexion produces a deep transgastric view of the tricuspid valve, which also permits optimal color flow and spectral Doppler evaluation of TR jets.

It is important at each level to rotate through multiple planes to comprehensively evaluate the TV and to use the simultaneous multiplane modality to help with identifying leaflets and appreciating adjacent anatomy. However, because of the variability of imaging planes as well as individual anatomy, leaflet identification should always be confirmed using the 3D en face view.

Three-Dimensional Echocardiography

Three-dimensional echocardiography obviates mental reconstruction of multiple 2D planes.[37] Lang and colleagues[33] suggested a standardized imaging display for the en face view of the TV with the interatrial septum placed inferiorly (at the 6-o'clock position) regardless of the atrial or ventricular orientation. Viewing the TV from the ventricular side (ie, TTE acquisition), the anterior leaflet would then be to the right and the posterior leaflet to the left. Viewing from the atrial side (ie, TEE acquisition), the anterior leaflet would then be to the left and the posterior leaflet to the right. Because of the anterior position of the right heart, 3D TTE images may be equal or sometimes better in quality compared with 3D TEE images. The current 3D systems have a different resolution for each of the 3 dimensions, with axial resolution (~0.5 mm) better than lateral (~2.5 mm) and elevational resolution (~3.0 mm).[37] Similar to 2D imaging, however, images in the far field may be subject to beam widening and attenuation. When creating 3D images, keep these current equipment limitations in mind realizing that optimal imaging of the TV may require an imaging plane between these standard windows. Obtaining multiple volumes from different views may still be necessary to fully characterize the valve and annulus. Finally, because of the complex nature of the valve, the volume acquired may need to have adjacent structures to help identify the leaflet anatomy, the aortic valve/aorta to identify the anterior leaflet, and the interatrial septum/mitral valve to identify the septal leaflet.

FLUOROSCOPIC ANATOMY OF THE TRICUSPID VALVE

Angiography and *fluoroscopy* have a complementary role in guiding procedural steps.

Interventional cardiologists are confident with the fluoroscopic anatomy of left-sided valves, unlike right-sided ones.[38] *Fluoroscopy* is useful in guiding device insertion into the right-sided chambers, orientation, and navigation toward the target zone. There are 2 perpendicular fluoroscopic working projections: the en face view of the valve, usually a left anterior oblique-caudal

projection, useful for navigating the catheter toward the target zone (similar to the 3D en face view but seen from the ventricular perspective), and the perpendicular valve plane view, usually a right anterior oblique-cranial projection useful to insert devices and catheters, to guide the trajectories and relations with TA and RV (similar to a 2-chamber view of the right heart).

In addition, angiography is fundamental for procedures targeting the annulus, in order to avoid potential coronary lesions due to the close relationship between the annulus and right coronary artery (RCA), especially in the septal and posterior portions. A good trick is to place a guidewire in the RCA in order to have a marker during the procedure.

COMPUTED TOMOGRAPHY

CT has an important role in preprocedural planning for TTVI, thanks to its high spatial and temporal resolution. The CT scan data set has to include the heart and angiography of the inferior and superior cava veins. CT imaging highlights target structures and also provides a vascular map, with complementary information to echocardiography and fluoroscopy, especially for transcatheter repair procedures targeting the annulus.

A CT scan provides information on annular structure and dilatation, the quality and the amount of annular tissue, and its relationship with the RCA in different regions. Another important aspect is a precise sizing of the IVC and its angle of insertion to the right atrium.

PREPROCEDURAL PLANNING OF PERCUTANEOUS TRICUSPID VALVE REPAIR

As for other transcatheter procedures, preprocedural planning and intraprocedural monitoring are fundamental. Preprocedural evaluation is focused on the selection of potential candidates and the selection of the most appropriate repair procedure or replacement.

The preprocedural planning is based on a multimodality imaging approach (**Table 1**), which aims to (1) define the mechanisms of TR; (2) characterize TV morphology; (3) analyze the anatomic relationships between the TV apparatus and other structures; and (4) determine the size of the inferior and superior vena cava.

A potential candidate for transcatheter correction of TR with plausible clinical benefit seems to be patients at high-prohibitive surgical risk, affected by FTR with normal TV leaflet morphology and excursion and predominant

Table 1
Multimodality imaging evaluation for tricuspid valve: preprocedural planning and intraprocedural monitoring

Imaging Modality	Applications	
	Preprocedural Setting	Intraprocedural Guidance
2D TTE or TEE	1. Anatomy of TV apparatus 2. Grading of TR and evaluation of area and gradients 3. TV remodeling parameters: annular dimensions, coaptation length and depth	1. Accurate visualization of devices 2. Guidance to the target zone and fine positioning of devices 3. Discerning annulus from leaflets 4. Assessment of angle of approach of device to the target
Simultaneous biplane view	Same as 2D views but with more accurate spatial localization	Same as 2D views but with more accurate spatial localization
3D TTE	1. Anatomy of TV apparatus 2. Grading of TR and area 3. More precise measurements of TV remodeling	Seldom used (see 3D TTE)
3D TEE	Same as 2D views; sometimes TEE has higher spatial resolution	1. Navigation of devices 2. Spatial relationships among structures
ICE		1. Navigation of devices 2. Guidance to the target zone and fine positioning of devices 3. Discerning annulus from leaflets
Fluoroscopy		1. Identification of catheters, guidewires, and other metallic devices 2. Rough navigation to the target zone
Angiography		1. Anatomic relationship of RCA
CT scan	1. TV remodeling parameters (TA shape, localization of commissures, accurate TA measurements) 2. Anatomic relationship of RCA 3. Semiquantitative evaluation of the tissue quality adjacent to the TA 4. Vascular map and IVC sizing	

Abbreviation: ICE, intracardiac echocardiography.

Adapted from Ancona F, Stella S, Taramasso M, et al. Multimodality imaging of the tricuspid valve with implication for percutaneous repair approaches. Heart 2017;103(14):1073–81; with permission.

annular dilatation, modest apical remodeling with at least preserved leaflet coaptation, without severe remodeling of the RV in terms of dilation and deterioration of systolic function, and pulmonary pressure not severely increased.[39] If TA dilation is the prevalent mechanism, techniques targeting the annulus emulating a surgical annuloplasty (Cardioband) or the Kay procedure (Trialign, TriCinch) seem to be the best choice. On the other hand, if there is no significant annular dilation (TA maximum diameter < 40 mm), leaflet coaptation is abnormal but preserved; if coaptation depth (CD) and coaptation length (CL)[34]

(CD < 11 mm, CL at least 2 mm)[40] between the target leaflets (usually septal and anterior) permit valid tissue grasping by a clip, the MitraClip System can be considered a suitable therapeutic option. In case of an extremely remodeled valve with a complete lack of coaptation or organic valve disease, the FORMA Spacer or TV replacement could be alternative options.

All potential candidates should be screened with TTE in order to evaluate all the previously mentioned features. If the eligibility of patients is confirmed, a second-level imaging evaluation with TEE and, in some cases, CT scan is mandatory in order to evaluate all of the anatomic details needed in the preprocedural setting. The quality of transesophageal and TTE is also an important limiting factor for intraprocedural monitoring.

INTRAPROCEDURAL IMAGING

A multimodality imaging approach (see **Table 1** for details) with 2D and 3D TEE, fluoroscopy, angiography, and intracardiac echocardiography (ICE) is used during percutaneous TV interventions.[41]

Two-dimensional and biplane views, because of superior spatial resolution, are best used for visualization of devices and their fine positioning as well as to evaluate TV remodeling parameters.

A 3D approach is of utmost importance to appreciate spatial relationships and guiding navigation. In order to customize the procedure, it is important to maintain the same 3D orientation all along the procedural steps: the authors' group has proposed the 3D surgical view, with the SVC at 11 o'clock and the IVC at 7 o'clock.[39]

TTE-based modalities could seldom be used for intraprocedural monitoring; because of its anterior position, the TV is well imaged by transthoracic examination. However, in the interventional arena, TTE is limited by the position of the patients and the position of the C-arm, requiring to temporarily stop the procedure.

Intraprocedural imaging, mainly by echocardiography, is essential to monitor each procedural step and to check the results; but it is also of paramount importance for early detection of potential catastrophic complications.

FUSION IMAGING

Fluoroscopy and echocardiography are the 2 imaging modalities used for intraprocedural monitoring and guidance. However, echocardiography provides high-resolution imaging of the soft tissues (leaflets, annulus, and so forth); but it is limited by artifacts in identifying metallic structures, such as guidewires and catheters, which are well defined on the fluoroscopic image. Moreover, echocardiography and fluoroscopy have their separate 3D coordinate spaces and display cardiac structures in different orientations. Thus, because of the technical complexity of transcatheter procedures, a better integration of echocardiography and fluoroscopic imaging is required.

A novel imaging technique (Echo-navigator, Philips Medical System, Best, The Netherlands) is able to acquire patient-specific imaging data from both fluoroscopic projections and 2D/3D TEE slices/perspectives and align them in the 3D space and in the time (**Figs. 1** and **2**).

Echocardiographic-fluoroscopic–fused imaging in TTVI could be useful to

- Better evaluate anatomic relationships
- Better localize the devices with easier navigation inside right-sided chambers
- Better assess trajectories and axial alignment of catheters and devices

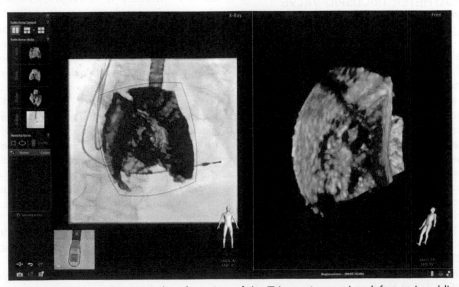

Fig. 1. Fusion imaging. Three-dimensional en face view of the TV superimposed on left anterior oblique caudal fluoroscopic projection. The fused image shows the en face view of the TV from the RV perspective.

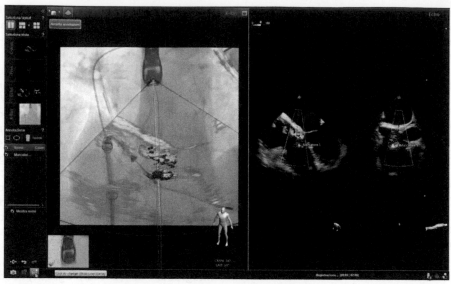

Fig. 2. Fusion imaging. A 2D color-Doppler 4-chamber view superimposed on left anterior oblique cranial fluoroscopic projection. The image shows the location of the regurgitant jet on the fluoroscopy.

- Localize the origin of the regurgitant jet on the fluoroscopic screen

The Echo-navigator system is limited, however, by the restricted rotation of the C-arm, which impedes some very useful 3D TEE perspectives to be merged with the fluoroscopic background. Another limitation is due to fiducial markers fixed on the screen and not exactly following soft tissue motion during cardiac cycle and respiratory movements.

TRANSCATHETER TRICUSPID VALVE INTERVENTIONS: DEVICES AND PROCEDURES

The Trialign system attempts to replicate the results of the Kay bicuspidization procedure, which has shown good mid-term and long-term[42] results. The system places pledgeted sutures within the TA spanning the length of the posterior leaflet and bicuspidizing the TV using a dedicated plication lock device to bring the 2 pledgeted sutures together. Since the first-in-human implantation of the Trialign system,[43] numerous other investigators have reported the successful use of this device for TR.[10,44] The Early Feasibility of the Mitralign Percutaneous Tricuspid Valve Annuloplasty System (PTVAS) (SCOUT) trial (ClinicalTrials.gov identifier: NCT02574650) has completed enrollment in the United States, and the CE mark trial in Europe (SCOUT II) has begun enrolling. The Trialign system (Fig. 3) uses a deflectable catheter

via the transjugular approach to deliver the device. The guide catheter and then the wire delivery catheter are positioned by echocardiographic guidance beneath the annulus, at the level of the postero-septal commissure. An insulated radiofrequency wire is used to cross the annulus with TEE imaging used to ensure adequate annular depth, away from the base of the leaflet and away from the right coronary artery. In order to image the wire crossing, multiple views can and typically should be used, including midesophageal views (typically at 60°–90° rotation) or transgastric views where the posterior annulus is in the near field. Implantation of the sutured pledget is performed using the wire as a catheter rail. After placement of the first pledget, a second wire/pledget is ideally positioned approximately 2.5 cm from the first catheter near the commissure between the posterior and anterior TV leaflets. The measurement of this distance can be performed along the curve of the annulus on 3D TEE images (either directly on the surgical view or on multi-planar reconstruction). Greater distances, particularly with a very curved posterior annulus, increase the stress on the annular tissue during plication and risk a pull-through (typically of a single pledget). A dedicated plication lock device is used to bring the two sutures together, plicating the annulus and effectively bicuspidizing the TV.

The Cardioband transcatheter system is currently indicated for the treatment of secondary (functional) mitral regurgitation (FMR). The

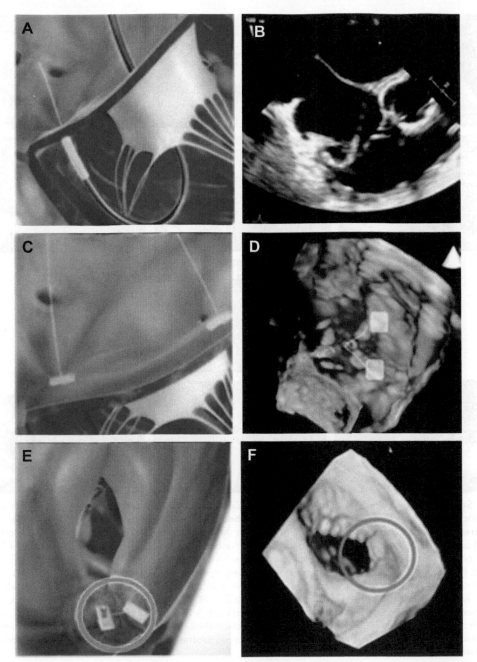

Fig. 3. Sequential intraprocedural imaging steps of the Mitralign procedure. The steps of the Mitralign include positioning the guide and wire delivery catheters below the posterior annulus (A, B) with echocardiographic guidance. After a second pledgeted suture is placed across the posterior annulus (C), they are drawn together (D) to plicate the annulus. Once maximally plicated, the pledgets are locked and the sutures cut (*blue circle* in E, F). In (F), using advanced photo-realistic 3D image rendering software, the pledgets and lock can be easily identified.

Cardioband (**Fig. 4**) is a direct annuloplasty transcatheter system, deployed on the beating heart through a transvenous approach. The implant is deployed along the posterior annulus of the mitral valve and is adjusted under transesophageal guidance on the beating heart.

Recent successes and European CE mark approval of the Cardioband system for FMR, which successfully reduced mitral regurgitation and was associated with improvement in heart failure symptoms as well as improvement in exercise capacity, demonstrated a favorable safety

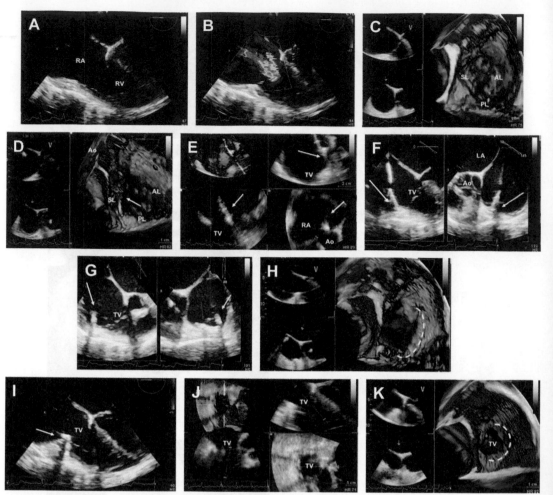

Fig. 4. Sequential intraprocedural imaging steps of the Cardioband procedure (part 1). Baseline evaluation at the beginning of the procedure: 2D midesophageal 4-chamber view (*A*) and 2D baseline color-Doppler (*B*). A 3D en face perspective of TV from the right atrium (RA) (*C*). The delivery system (*arrow*) is advanced and steered toward the first target site (in this case at the antero-septal commissure area) ([*D*] 3D en face perspective view of TV). Precise tip positioning of the delivery catheter (*arrows*) on the TA is imaged by multiplanar reconstruction (*E*) or simultaneous biplane view (*F*). Sequential intraprocedural imaging steps of Cardioband procedure (part 2). The first procedural steps are repeated for every implanted screw: the band (*red arrow*) and the delivery catheter (*white arrows*) are visualized under simultaneous biplane view (*G*). A 3D en face perspective view (*H*) allows evaluation of the band positioning along leaflet hinge points (*dotted line*). A 2D midesophageal 4-chamber view (*I, white arrow* points toward the device) and multiplanar reconstruction showing TA reduction (*J*). A 3D en face perspective view (*K*) allows for final result evaluation and band positioning (*dotted arrow*). AL, anterior leaflet; Ao, aortic valve; LA, left atrium; PL, posterior leaflet; SL, septal leaflet.

profile (no periprocedural deaths).[45] In this setting, several of these investigators successfully performed a modification of this procedure for FTR showing reductions in annular dimensions, regurgitant volume, regurgitant orifice areas, and mean right atrial pressures. The Cardioband implant is a polyester sleeve with radiopaque markers spaced 8 mm apart. The sleeve covers the delivery system that deploys anchors guided by TEE. A contraction wire is premounted on the Cardioband sleeve, and

contracting the polyester sleeve from one side is accomplished using a dedicated cinching tool and results in a proportional reduction of the distances between the implanted anchors and significant annular remodeling.[46] The TRI-REPAIR-CE trial is now enrolling in France, Germany, and Italy (ClinicalTrials.gov identifier: NCT02981953).

The *FORMA Spacer* device (**Fig. 5**) is implanted from a left subclavian vein approach, introducing an anchor, attached to a

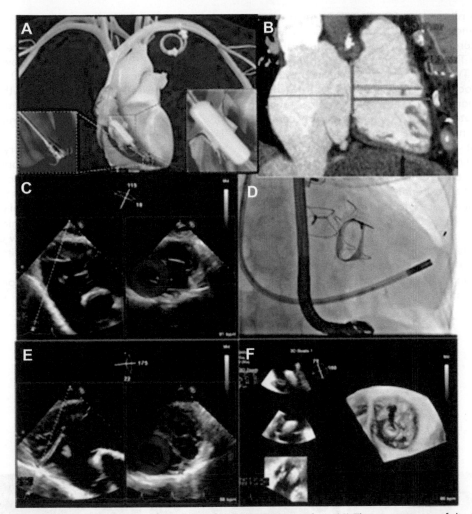

Fig. 5. Sequential intraprocedural imaging steps of the FORMA procedure. (A) The components of the FORMA device: anchor (*left insert*) and the spacer device (*right insert*). (B) The preprocedural CT measurement of RV height in diastole. (C) The intraprocedural transgastric biplane image with ideal position of the anchor and (D) The positioning of the anchor on fluoroscopy. (E) The final position of the anchor (*blue line, blue star*). The final position can be adjusted using 3D imaging (F).

foam-filled spacer device, which then forms a surface against which the leaflet tips coapt. Since the early report of 7 successful implants in high-risk patients with severe TR with no procedural complications,[13] the US early feasibility trial was begun (ClinicalTrials.gov identifier: NCT02471807) and is currently enrolling. Two sizes of the spacer device are currently available, 12 mm and 15 mm diameter, with the device choice determined by the largest echocardiographic vena contracta width. Preprocedural planning is essential, using CT to determine the complex anatomy of the RV (ie, location of trabeculations, moderator band, and papillary muscle). Intraprocedural imaging relies heavily on both intraprocedural fluoroscopic and 2D/3D TEE guidance. The initial preimplantation

TEE imaging should include (1) the identification of the ideal landing zone of the RV anchor (corresponding to the position on CT); (2) imaging of the path of the anchor within the RV to assess for possible impediments to positioning (ie, papillary muscles, trabeculations, or moderator band); and (3) the location and severity of TR to aid in optimal positioning of the device. During implantation, TEE is ideal for (1) guiding the balloon-tip catheter to the ideal location for the anchor position; (2) confirming the unimpeded path of the device catheter sweep from the posterior to anterior annulus; (3) anchor deployment into the RV myocardium with a tug test to ensure stable device implantation and the absence of pericardial effusion; and (4) positioning of the device to optimize the reduction in TR. After device placement, 2D/3D TTE imaging can be performed to assess the final position and 3D vena contracta area (VCS) of the residual jets.

The *TriCinch System* is a dedicated percutaneous TV repair device that mimics the surgical Kay procedure by cinching the TA at the anteroposterior commissure (APC), thus, reducing the septolateral TA dimensions and, therefore, improving leaflet coaptation. A corkscrew implant is permanently placed, and a self-expanding stent is deployed in the hepatic region of the IVC to apply tension (**Fig. 6**). After the initial experience,[8,9,47] the Percutaneous Treatment of Tricuspid Valve Regurgitation With the TriCinch System (PREVENT) trial (ClinicalTrials.gov identifier: NCT02098200) has completed enrollment in Europe.

At the beginning of the procedure in the catheterization laboratory, under deep sedation or general anesthesia, a baseline careful evaluation of the degree of TR, dimensions of TA, and CL has to be performed. The procedure starts by placing the guidewire in the RV, a step monitored by 2D TEE, also using biplane views, starting from a midesophageal view of 30° to 70°. After guidewire placement, the catheter is inserted and advanced into the right atrium (the 3D surgical view permits locating the system inside the right heart chambers).

The next step is to guide the delivery system to the target site (usually the anteroposterior commissure, the third segment): A complete and accurate spatial visualization of all structures at the same time (leaflets, annulus, atrial wall and IVC junction) is achieved by the 3D surgical view, following the steering of the corkscrew delivery system toward the third segment and its subsequent advancement to contact the annulus. Biplane view monitors fine-tip positioning on the annulus, accurately discerning it from

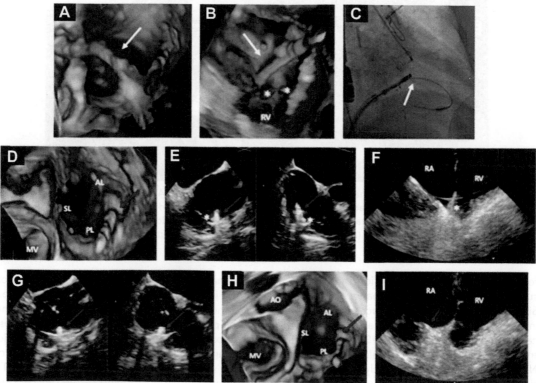

Fig. 6. Sequential intraprocedural imaging steps of TriCinch procedure (part 1). The guidewire (*arrow*) is advanced into right chambers toward TV (*asterisks:* valve leaflets) under 3D surgical view of right atrium (RA) (*A*) and 3D lateral perspective of RV (*B*). Fluoroscopy could be useful, highlighting the device (*arrow*) in RA (left anterior oblique view [*C*]). The corkscrew delivery system (*arrow*) is advanced and steered toward the target site (in this case at the APC area) ([*D*] 3D en face perspective view of TV). Precise tip positioning of the delivery catheter (*arrow*) on the TA (*asterisks*) is imaged by multiplanar reconstruction or simultaneous biplane view (*E*). ICE could be very useful in discerning leaflets from TA (*asterisk*), showing the tip of delivery catheter (*arrow*) (*F*). After implantation, a pull test of the system (*arrow*) is visualized under simultaneous biplane view (*G*) and ICE imaging (*I*). A 3D en face perspective view (*H*) allows for final result evaluation, after corkscrew implantation (*arrow*) and stent deployment. AL, Anterior Leaflet; AO, aortic valve; MV, mitral valve; PL, posterior leaflet; SL, septal leaflet.

leaflets, assessing the local angle of approach and optimally visualizing guidewire, catheter, and corkscrew. At this point, ICE imaging can be very helpful.

A recheck of the final location of the corkscrew and its relation with the RCA is fundamental, with biplane and 3D views, together with angiographic imaging of the RCA. If the positioning is correct and there is no risk for coronary lesions, the screw is inserted.

After corkscrew implantation, a pull test is performed under direct TEE evaluation in multiple or better biplane views, checking the results of the applied tension and its maintenance. Before the final cinching of the system, a 3D view of the valve to assess the remodeling parameters and a transvalvular gradient are acquired to have a baseline for subsequent steps.

In fact, before and after each degree of cinching, a color-Doppler evaluation together with measurements of annulus diameters, CL, TV area, and TR severity are needed.

The cinching of the TA is finally maintained by implantation of a self-expanding stent in the IVC. About 10 minutes after stent deployment, a final recheck assessing changes of residual jet geometry, new jet occurrence, leaflet integrity, and importantly possible fatal complications, such as pericardial effusion or new wall motion abnormalities in the RCA territory, is performed.

The *MitraClip System*, conceived for percutaneous mitral repair, is also an appealing percutaneous solution in case of FTR with suitable anatomy.[48] This approach aims to increase leaflet coaptation, mimicking a sort of zip mechanism between 2 out of 3 TV leaflets (**Fig. 7**).

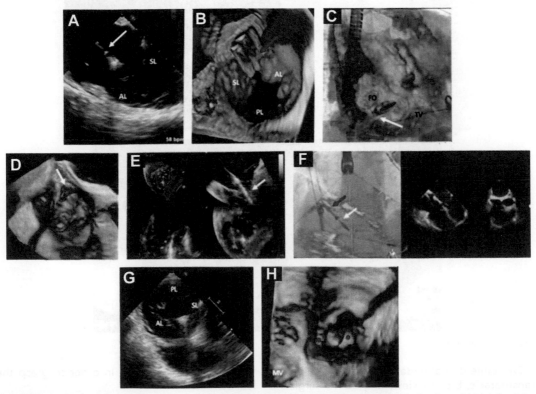

Fig. 7. Sequential intraprocedural imaging steps of the MitraClip procedure (part 1). Navigation within right atrium (RA) toward TV: guide catheter (GC; *red arrow*) and mitraclip delivery system (*white arrow*) are first advanced inside RA (A) 2D midesophageal 4-chamber view; (B) 3D en face perspective view; (C) fusion imaging on fluoroscopic right anterior oblique (RAO) projection. Definition of delivery system trajectory: GC (*red arrow*) and MDS (*white arrow*) approaching TV (D) 3D oblique perspective view; (E) multiplanar reconstruction; (F) fusion imaging on fluoroscopic antero-posterior projection. Sequential intraprocedural imaging steps of the MitraClip procedure (part 2). The first clip arms (*asterisks*) are orientated perpendicular to the coaptation line between AL and SL ([G] transgastric short axis view, [H] 3D en face perspective view). The clip (*arrow*) is finally implanted and released ([I] 2D transgastric short axis view; [J] 3D en face view from the RA). The second clip with opened arms (*arrows*) is advanced into the RV below TV leaflets ([K] fusion imaging: simultaneous biplane view and its superimposition on fluoroscopic RAO view). TV leaflets are then captured (*red arrow:* clip closed) ([L] simultaneous biplane view). AO, aortic valve; FO, foramen ovale. MV, mitral valve.

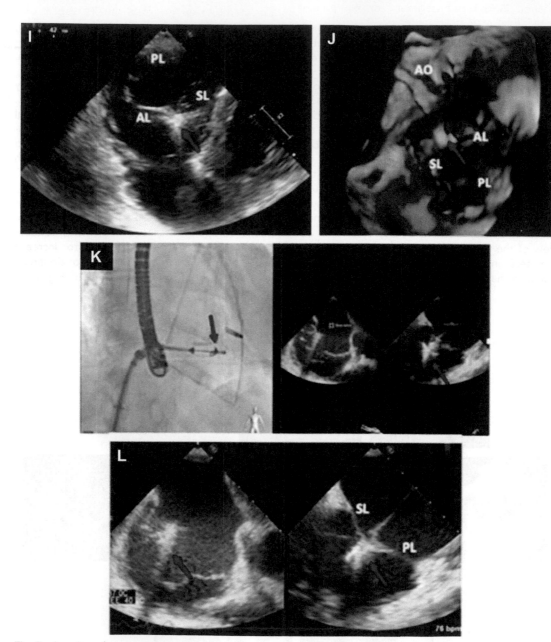

Fig. 7. (continued)

Two-dimensional midesophageal, or seldom transthoracic, biplane views and 3D TV surgical views enable guiding the correct position of the delivery catheter targeting the main regurgitant lesion, with the MitraClip arms perpendicular to the line of coaptation of the 2 leaflets. 3D TEE guides clockwise or counter-clockwise orientation of the clip arms to ensure a perpendicular orientation with respect to the leaflets. Fusion imaging could help for this purpose, getting the trajectory easier for the interventionalist. The MitraClip is then advanced across the valve and gradually pulled back from the ventricular side in order to grasp the leaflets.

Two-dimensional midesophageal biplane views and transgastric short-axis views are of the utmost importance for this procedural step. Once the clip position is optimized, the grippers are dropped and the clip arms are closed. The implantation result can be clearly seen in 2D transgastric TV short axis and in 3D reconstructions. If significant TR remains and no significant tricuspid stenosis is observed, additional clips may be placed at the area of greatest residual regurgitation, in a sort of zip

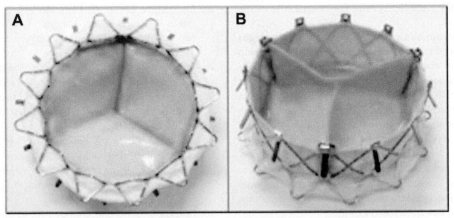

Fig. 8. The GATE valve. The GATE tricuspid atrioventricular valved stent (atrial side in [A] and ventricular side in [B]). (*Courtesy of* NaviGate Cardiac Structures Inc, Lake Forest, CA; with permission).

fashion. In cases of complete zipping of one commissure, the final result could be the bicuspidization of the TV.

A transcatheter TV device, the *GATE Tricuspid Atrioventricular Valved Stent* (NaviGate Cardiac Structures Inc, Lake Forest, CA) (**Fig. 8**), has recently been implanted in 3 high-risk patients. This device can be implanted by a transjugular or transatrial approach. A pigtail catheter is positioned in the RV for periodic ventriculography. A right coronary artery wire is placed in the distal artery to help identify the annular plane and guide valve placement. Alignment of the valve is easily performed on fluoroscopy by aligning marker lines on the capsule in a right anterior oblique view. Fine adjustments of positioning are performed before the final release using fluoroscopy or TEE; in some instances, ICE imaging may be useful. The anchoring and left ventricular outflow tract obstruction issues of transcatheter mitral valve replacement are not shared on the right side, and this device may have great utility not only with FTR but also with degenerative disease. The assessment of residual para-valvular regurgitation is performed using color-Doppler echocardiography; however, cardiac MRI or 3D echocardiography to quantify the total RV stroke volume and then subtract the forward stroke volume to measure regurgitant volume may be useful.

REFERENCES

1. Agricola E, Stella S, Gullace M, et al. Impact of functional tricuspid regurgitation on heart failure and death in patients with functional mitral regurgitation and left ventricular dysfunction. Eur J Heart Fail 2012;14(8):902–8.

2. Arsalan M, Walther T, Smith RL 2nd, et al. Tricuspid regurgitation diagnosis and treatment. Eur Heart J 2017;38(9):634–8.

3. Topilsky Y, Khanna AD, Oh JK, et al. Preoperative factors associated with adverse outcome after tricuspid valve replacement. Circulation 2011; 123(18):1929–39.

4. Agarwal S, Tuzcu EM, Rodriguez ER, et al. Interventional cardiology perspective of functional tricuspid regurgitation. Circ Cardiovasc Interv 2009;2(6):565–73.

5. McElhinney DB, Cabalka AK, Aboulhosn JA, et al. Transcatheter tricuspid valve-in-valve implantation for the treatment of dysfunctional surgical bioprosthetic valves: an international, multicenter registry study. Circulation 2016;133(16):1582–93.

6. Cabasa AS, Eleid MF, Rihal CS, et al. Tricuspid valve replacement: a percutaneous transfemoral valve-in-ring approach. JACC Cardiovasc Interv 2015;8(8):1126–8.

7. Lauten A, Doenst T, Hamadanchi A, et al. Percutaneous bicaval valve implantation for transcatheter treatment of tricuspid regurgitation: clinical observations and 12-month follow-up. Circ Cardiovasc Interv 2014;7(2):268–72.

8. Latib A, Agricola E, Pozzoli A, et al. First-in-man implantation of a tricuspid annular remodeling device for functional tricuspid regurgitation. JACC Cardiovasc Interv 2015;8(13):e211–4.

9. Latib A, Mangieri A, Vicentini L, et al. Percutaneous tricuspid valve annuloplasty under conscious sedation (with only fluoroscopic and intracardiac echocardiography monitoring). JACC Cardiovasc Interv 2017;10(6):620–1.

10. Latib A, Ancona MB, Agricola E, et al. Percutaneous bicuspidization of the tricuspid valve. JACC Cardiovasc Imaging 2017;10(4):488–9.

11. Hammerstingl C, Schueler R, Malasa M, et al. Transcatheter treatment of severe tricuspid regurgitation

with the MitraClip system. Eur Heart J 2016;37(10): 849–53.

12. Taramasso M, Latib A, Denti P, et al. Percutaneous repair of the tricuspid valve using a novel cinching device: acute and chronic experience in a preclinical large animal model. EuroIntervention 2016; 12(7):918–25.

13. Campelo-Parada F, Perlman G, Philippon F, et al. First-in-man experience of a novel transcatheter repair system for treating severe tricuspid regurgitation. J Am Coll Cardiol 2015;66(22):2475–83.

14. Bai Y, Zong GJ, Wang HR, et al. An integrated pericardial valved stent special for percutaneous tricuspid implantation: an animal feasibility study. J Surg Res 2010;160(2):215–21.

15. Anwar AM, Geleijnse ML, Soliman OI, et al. Assessment of normal tricuspid valve anatomy in adults by real-time three-dimensional echocardiography. Int J Cardiovasc Imaging 2007;23(6):717–24.

16. Martinez RM, O'Leary PW, Anderson RH. Anatomy and echocardiography of the normal and abnormal tricuspid valve. Cardiol Young 2006;16(Suppl 3): 4–11.

17. Fukuda S, Saracino G, Matsumura Y, et al. Three-dimensional geometry of the tricuspid annulus in healthy subjects and in patients with functional tricuspid regurgitation: a real-time, 3-dimensional echocardiographic study. Circulation 2006;114(1 Suppl):I492–8.

18. Mahmood F, Kim H, Chaudary B, et al. Tricuspid annular geometry: a three-dimensional transesophageal echocardiographic study. J Cardiothorac Vasc Anesth 2013;27(4):639–46.

19. Addetia K, Yamat M, Mediratta A, et al. Comprehensive two-dimensional interrogation of the tricuspid valve using knowledge derived from three-dimensional echocardiography. J Am Soc Echocardiography 2015;29(1):74–82.

20. Ton-Nu TT, Levine RA, Handschumacher MD, et al. Geometric determinants of functional tricuspid regurgitation: insights from 3-dimensional echocardiography. Circulation 2006;114(2):143–9.

21. Huu N, Monod-Nguyen B, Vallée J, et al. Anatomical relations of the atrio-ventricular junction (anuli fibrosi atrioventricularis). Anatomia Clinica 1982; 3(4):339–55.

22. Wafae N, Hayashi H, Gerola LR, et al. Anatomical study of the human tricuspid valve. Surg Radiol Anat 1990;12(1):37–41.

23. Nigri GR, Di Dio LJ, Baptista CA. Papillary muscles and tendinous cords of the right ventricle of the human heart: morphological characteristics. Surg Radiol Anat 2001;23(1):45–9.

24. Tretter JT, Sarwark AE, Anderson RH, et al. Assessment of the anatomical variation to be found in the normal tricuspid valve. Clin Anat 2016;29(3): 399–407.

25. Nemoto N, Lesser JR, Pedersen WR, et al. Pathogenic structural heart changes in early tricuspid regurgitation. J Thorac Cardiovasc Surg 2015; 150(2):323–30.

26. Spinner EM, Buice D, Yap CH, et al. The effects of a three-dimensional, saddle-shaped annulus on anterior and posterior leaflet stretch and regurgitation of the tricuspid valve. Ann Biomed Eng 2012; 40(5):996–1005.

27. Topilsky Y, Khanna A, Le Tourneau T, et al. Clinical context and mechanism of functional tricuspid regurgitation in patients with and without pulmonary hypertension. Circ Cardiovasc Imaging 2012; 5(3):314–23.

28. Fukuda S, Song JM, Gillinov AM, et al. Tricuspid valve tethering predicts residual tricuspid regurgitation after tricuspid annuloplasty. Circulation 2005;111(8):975–9.

29. Park YH, Song JM, Lee EY, et al. Geometric and hemodynamic determinants of functional tricuspid regurgitation: a real-time three-dimensional echocardiography study. Int J Cardiol 2008;124(2): 160–5.

30. Rudski LG, Lai WW, Afilalo J, et al. Guidelines for the echocardiographic assessment of the right heart in adults: a report from the American Society of Echocardiography endorsed by the European Association of Echocardiography, a registered branch of the European Society of Cardiology, and the Canadian Society of Echocardiography. J Am Soc Echocardiography 2010;23(7):685–713 [quiz: 786–8].

31. Lang RM, Badano LP, Mor-Avi V, et al. Recommendations for cardiac chamber quantification by echocardiography in adults: an update from the American Society of Echocardiography and the European Association of Cardiovascular Imaging. J Am Soc Echocardiography 2015;28(1):1–39.e14.

32. Hahn RT, Abraham T, Adams MS, et al. Guidelines for performing a comprehensive transesophageal echocardiographic examination: recommendations from the American Society of Echocardiography and the Society of Cardiovascular Anesthesiologists. J Am Soc Echocardiogr 2013;26(9):921–64.

33. Lang RM, Badano LP, Tsang W, et al. EAE/ASE recommendations for image acquisition and display using three-dimensional echocardiography. J Am Soc Echocardiography 2012;25(1):3–46.

34. Stankovic I, Daraban AM, Jasaityte R, et al. Incremental value of the en face view of the tricuspid valve by two-dimensional and three-dimensional echocardiography for accurate identification of tricuspid valve leaflets. J Am Soc Echocardiography 2014;27(4):376–84.

35. Chan KL, Veinot JP. Anatomic basis of echocardiographic diagnosis. , London: Springer; 2011. p. xiv, 491.

36. Otto CM. Textbook of clinical echocardiography. 5th edition. Philadelphia: Elsevier/Saunders; 2013.

37. Badano LP, Agricola E, Perez de Isla L, et al. Evaluation of the tricuspid valve morphology and function by transthoracic real-time three-dimensional echocardiography. Eur J Echocardiography 2009; 10(4):477–84.

38. Theriault-Lauzier P, Andalib A, Martucci G, et al. Fluoroscopic anatomy of left-sided heart structures for transcatheter interventions: insight from multi-slice computed tomography. JACC Cardiovasc Interv 2014;7(9):947–57.

39. Ancona F, Stella S, Taramasso M, et al. Multimodality imaging of the tricuspid valve with implication for percutaneous repair approaches. Heart 2017; 103(14):1073–81.

40. Attizzani GF, Ohno Y, Capodanno D, et al. Extended use of percutaneous edge-to-edge mitral valve repair beyond EVEREST (Endovascular Valve Edge-to-Edge Repair) criteria: 30-day and 12-month clinical and echocardiographic outcomes from the GRASP (Getting Reduction of Mitral Insufficiency by Percutaneous Clip Implantation) registry. JACC Cardiovasc Interv 2015;8(1 Pt A):74–82.

41. Agricola E, Ancona F, Stella S, et al. Use of echocardiography for guiding percutaneous tricuspid valve procedures. JACC Cardiovasc Imaging 2017;10(10 Pt A):1194–8.

42. Taramasso M, Vanermen H, Maisano F, et al. The growing clinical importance of secondary tricuspid regurgitation. J Am Coll Cardiol 2012;59(8):703–10.

43. Schofer J, Bijuklic K, Tiburtius C, et al. First-in-human transcatheter tricuspid valve repair in a patient with severely regurgitant tricuspid valve. J Am Coll Cardiol 2015;65(12):1190–5.

44. Malasa M, Werner N, Nickenig G, et al. Transcatheter tricuspid valve repair in a patient with isolated functional tricuspid valve regurgitation. Eur Heart J 2016;37(10):855.

45. Nickenig G, Hammerstingl C, Schueler R, et al. Transcatheter mitral annuloplasty in chronic functional mitral regurgitation: 6-month results with the cardioband percutaneous mitral repair system. JACC Cardiovasc Interv 2016;9(19):2039–47.

46. Arsalan M, Agricola E, Alfieri O, et al. Effect of transcatheter mitral annuloplasty with the cardioband device on 3-dimensional geometry of the mitral annulus. Am J Cardiol 2016;118(5): 744–9.

47. Rosser BA, Taramasso M, Maisano F. Transcatheter interventions for tricuspid regurgitation: TriCinch (4Tech). EuroIntervention 2016;12(Y):Y110–2.

48. Nickenig G, Kowalski M, Hausleiter J, et al. Transcatheter treatment of severe tricuspid regurgitation with the edge-to-edge mitraclip technique. Circulation 2017;135(19):1802–14.

Percutaneous Tricuspid Annuloplasty

Antonio Mangieri, MD[a],*, Scott Lim, MD[b], Jason H. Rogers, MD[c], Azeem Latib, MD, FESC[a]

KEYWORDS

• Tricuspid regurgitation • Right-sided heart failure • Tricuspid annuloplasty

---

KEY POINTS

- The tricuspid valve was ignored for a long time.
- The prevalence of severe tricuspid regurgitation, however, is not negligible and is associated with poor prognosis.
- In cases of primary tricuspid regurgitation, surgical options are limited by a high risk of mortality and morbidity.
- New percutaneous approaches are becoming available to meet this consistent unmet clinical need.
- This review presents the current available devices that reproduce both the complete and uncomplete surgical annuloplasty techniques.

INTRODUCTION

Functional tricuspid regurgitation (FTR) represents the most frequent type of tricuspid regurgitation (TR) encountered, whereas TR caused by primary (organic) valve lesions is uncommon.[1] FTR (also known as secondary TR) can be the result of left-sided valvular or myocardial dysfunction or of pulmonary hypertension in absence of organic disease of the tricuspid valve.[2] In approximately 20% of cases, FTR is secondary to a primary dilation of the right atrium and/or ventricle. The final common pathway resulting in FTR is invariably tricuspid annular dilatation that occurs mainly in the posterior and anterior parts of the valve (along the right ventricular free wall). When annular dilation occurs, the annulus loses its usual saddle shape and becomes flattened. The enlargement of the right ventricle and tricuspid annulus creates the anatomic basis of TR due to the lack of leaflet coaptation.[3] In the

advanced stage of the disease, worsening of the TR is caused by a progressive increase in the annular and right ventricular chamber diameters. When this occurs, reducing the tricuspid annular diameter with annuloplasty has been the primary target in the surgical treatment of FTR.[4] Many patients suffering from severe TR, however, remain untreated because of prohibitive surgical risk. In this setting, emerging percutaneous tricuspid annuloplasty devices have been developed to satisfy this unmet clinical need.

SURGICAL BACKGROUND

The surgical repair of TR secondary to annular dilation can be performed using 2 surgical methods: (1) suture annuloplasty and (2) ring annuloplasty.[5]

The purpose of suture annuloplasty is to reduce annular dimensions by using a surgical suture technique (usually with pledgets) to

---

Disclosures: None.
[a] Interventional Cardiology Unit, IRCCS San Raffaele Scientific Institute, Via Olgettina 60, Milan 20132, Italy; [b] Department of Cardiology, University of Virginia, 1215 Lee Street, Charlottesville, VA 22903, USA; [c] Division of Cardiovascular Medicine, UC Davis Medical Center, 2315 Stockton Boulevard, Sacramento, CA 95817, USA
* Corresponding author. Interventional Cardiology Unit, IRCCS San Raffaele Scientific Institute, Via Olgettina 60, Milan 20132, Italy.
E-mail address: antonio.mangieri@gmail.com

Intervent Cardiol Clin 7 (2018) 31–36
https://doi.org/10.1016/j.iccl.2017.08.006

purse-string the annulus. Most suture annuloplasty techniques replicate either the technique popularized by Taramasso and colleagues[6] or the De Vega annuloplasty. The Kay annuloplasty technique results in bicuspidization of the tricuspid valve by plicating the posterior leaflet. The De Vega technique is based on suturing the annulus surrounding the anterior and the posterior leaflets, improving leaflet coaptation. The durability of suture annuloplasty is limited, however, due to inadequate or recurrent annular dilation, which can be related to suture dehiscence due to the presence of friable tissue.

Ring annuloplasty consists of the implantation of a prosthetic annuloplasty ring. Rigid rings are able to effectively reduce the tricuspid annular diameter and improve leaflet coaptation and have been shown more durable than suture-based annuloplasty in surgical series. Some rings can also restore the native 3-D shape of the tricuspid annulus. A rigid ring can interfere, however, with the physiologic systolic and diastolic excursion of the tricuspid annulus during the cardiac cycle.[7] Flexible bands have an adaptive movement in synergy with tricuspid annulus excursion but have worse results in terms of TR recurrence.[8]

ANATOMIC CHALLENGES FOR PERCUTANEOUS TRICUSPID ANNULOPLASTY

Several percutaneous annuloplasty systems are based on established surgical techniques. These percutaneous technologies address the predominant pathophysiologic mechanism of FTR, which is annular dilatation. Several anatomic factors may represent a challenge, however, for the percutaneous treatment of FTR[9]:

- The target zone for percutaneous tricuspid annuloplasty is the anterolateral part of the tricuspid annulus, which is in close proximity with the right coronary artery (RCA).[10]
- Few percutaneous routes are available to achieve an ideal approach for the percutaneous treatment of the tricuspid valve. The thin wall of the right ventricle does not allow the transapical approach. The transfemoral venous route is limited by the frequently unfavorable angle between the tricuspid annulus and inferior vena cava. Access from the internal jugular vein or superior vena cava has a more favorable approach angle to the tricuspid valve, but gaining access in the neck can be ergonomically awkward in the catheter laboratory environment. The small subvalvular space and the high number of trabeculae limit the possible movements below the valvular plane.
- Due to large native tricuspid annular diameters, the introducer sheath and the delivery system need to accommodate a prosthesis approximately twice the size of the prostheses used for transcatheter aortic valve replacement.
- Lack of widespread knowledge on the performance of standardized imaging required for the interventional guidance of transcatheter tricuspid procedures. Transesophageal echocardiography is limited by the anterior location of the valve. 2-D echo has the limitation that it can rarely visualize the 3 leaflets together. Moreover, the esophagus is not axial with nor in close proximity to the tricuspid valve so midesophageal images are off-axis and, therefore, more challenging to orient. 3-D echocardiography has overcome this problem by giving simultaneous visualization of the 3 leaflets; however, poor acoustic windows in some patients and a lack of standardization of imaging views is a major limitation.[11] There is limited experience with the use of intracardiac echocardiography, although this has the advantage of being in the right atrium and can provide highly detailed imaging if aligned correctly.
- Current devices dedicated to percutaneous tricuspid annuloplasty require a certain amount of space between the RCA and the tricuspid annulus (to avoid injuring the RCA) as well as a good tissue quality.[12]
- The tricuspid valve and annulus poses several anatomic challenges. The contemporary available devices for percutaneous tricuspid annuloplasty require good-quality tissue and enough space between the tricuspid annulus and the RCA to be safely implanted. The late device detachments and tissue dehiscence that occurred after first percutaneous experiences can be a consequence of tissue fragility that limist safe and prolonged anchoring of the devices.[13]

PERCUTANEOUS ANNULOPLASTY SYSTEMS FOR TRICUSPID REGURGITATION

The currently available percutaneous tricuspid annuloplasty systems can be categorized as follows:

- Complete percutaneous tricuspid annuloplasty systems: Cardioband (Edwards Lifesciences, Irvine, CA), IRIS (Millipede, Santa Rosa, CA), Minimally Invasive Annuloplasty (MIA) (Micro Interventional Devices, Inc, Newtown, PA), and Transatrial intrapericardial tricuspid annuloplasty (TRAIPTA)
- Incomplete percutaneous tricuspid annuloplasty systems: TriCinch System (4Tech, Galway, Ireland) and Trialign (Mitralign, Tewksbury, Massachussetts)

A brief description of the devices is reported in **Fig. 1**. The complete annuloplasty devices reproduce surgical ring annuloplasty and theoretically could have better long-term durability with less recurrence of significant TR. Few clinical experiences have been reported, however, and little is known about the efficacy and durability of such procedures. Greater clinical experience is available regarding incomplete percutaneous tricuspid annuloplasty systems. These devices may potentially be less effective, however, in the long term in preventing the recurrence of significant TR, especially in patients marked annular dilatation and/or tricuspid valve tenting.

Cardioband

The Cardioband system is a direct surgical-like annuloplasty device commercially available for the treatment of functional mitral regurgitation. The band has different sizes and is inserted through a 24-French (Fr) sheath placed in the femoral vein with a similar delivery system to that used for other mitral procedures.[14] The Cardioband can also be used for FTR and once the anchors are fixed around the annulus, the band is cinched, obtaining a controlled reduction of the anteroposterior and septolateral dimensions of the tricuspid valve. The tricuspid Cardioband has been implanted under compassionate use in 5 patients with satisfying results. The investigators report a 23% to 45% reduction of the annular dimensions, 50% to 70% reduction of effective regurgitant orifice area without any serious adverse event occurred during the procedures.[15] The European Conformité Européenne (CE) mark study (TrIcuspid Regurgitation RePAIr With CaRdioband Transcatheter System [TRI-REPAIR]) is recruiting patients with FTR and annular diameter greater than 40 mm. The first patient enrolled in the study had significant hemodynamic improvement post-cinching, including a reduction in TR grade (from severe to mild), reductions in septolateral and anteroposterior diameter (42.2% and 25%, respectively), proximal isovelocity surface area radius (50%), and vena contracta (46.9%).

IRIS

The IRIS is a complete, adjustable, semirigid annuloplasty ring. The device is fully

	Trialign	Tricinch	MIA	Cardioband	Millipede	Traipta
Device name and structure	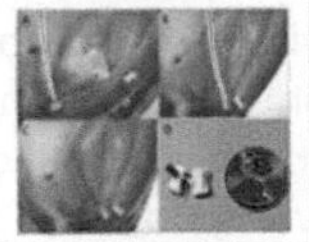	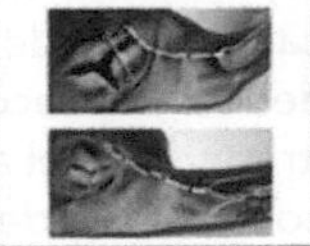	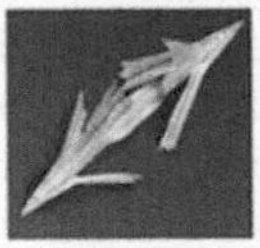	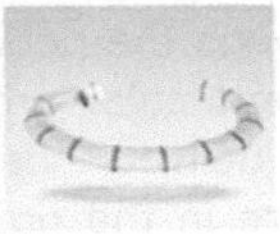	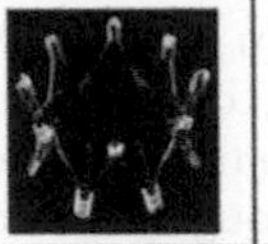	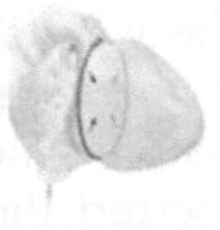
Type of annuloplasty	Incomplete annuloplasty	Incomplete annuloplasty	Complete annuloplasty	Complete annuloplasty	Complete annuloplasty	Complete annuloplasty
Study (ClinicalTrials.gov identifier)	SCOUT I (NCT02574650) SCOUT II (not registered)	PREVENT (NCT02098200)	STTAR (not registred)	TRI-REPAIR (NCT02981953)	No study available	No study available
Clinical experiences	15 patients enrolled in the SCOUT I 14 patients treated for compassionate use	24 patients treated in the PREVENT study	2 surgical implants	30 patients enrolled in the TRI-REPAIR study 5 patients treated for compassionate use	9 surgical implants	No clinical data available Pre clinical implants in 16 swine
Adverse events	3 single-pledget annular detachments 1 right coronary stenting	4 late anchor detachment 2 haemopericardium	Not reported	Not reported	Not reported	1 moderate pericardial effusion

Fig. 1. Transcatheter therapies for treating functional tricuspid valve regurgitation.

repositionable and retrievable prior to final deployment and can be used for the treatment of both mitral and TR without precluding future percutaneous options, such as edge-to-edge repair. IRIS has been used in 9 surgical patients between. In 2 cases the IRIS was implanted on both the mitral and tricuspid valve. Both patients experienced a reduction in TR severity with a reduction in tricuspid annulus diameter of 42% to 45% and final TR grade zero.[16] The percutaneous delivery of the IRIS has recently been performed successfully for the treatment of functional MR in human subjects. A transcatheter delivery system for the tricuspid IRIS is currently under clinical development.

MINIMALLY INVASIVE ANNULOPLASTY

The MIA device reduces tricuspid annular dimensions without sutures or other intervention due to the compliant, self-tensioning MIA implant incorporating the company's proprietary PolyCor anchors and MyoLast implantable elastomer. The 16F steerable delivery system has an end effector, which allows the deployment of the device in a 270° partial ring pattern. The two first in-human implants have been recently performed obtaining a significant reduction of the tricuspid valve area without any adverse events. The Study of Transcatheter Tricuspid Annular Repair (STTAR) trial will evaluate the performance of the MIA device in 40 patients with FTR.

Transatrial intrapericardial tricuspid annuloplasty

Transatrial intrapericardial tricuspid annulopasty (TRAIPTA) is an indirect transcatheter annuloplasty system inserted through the pericardium at the level of the atrioventricular groove. A custom memory-shaped delivery device is inserted through a puncture in the right atrial appendage. The implant is premounted on the delivery device loop and is preloaded into a 12F braided sheath. A circumferential suture is adjusted according to the dimension of the tricuspid annulus. An occluder is then placed in the right appendage to close the access to the pericardial space. Preclinical data from 16 swine showed good safety profile and efficacy: 1 moderate pericardial effusion without tamponade occurred and no other complications were described. The device was effective in the reduction of the septolateral (49%) and anteroposterior (31%) dimensions of the tricuspid annulus. Cook Medical (Bloomington, Indiana, United States) is developing TRAIPTA for human use. The main limitation of the device is the inability

to treat patients with previous cardiac surgery due to adhesions in the pericardial space.[17]

TriCinch System

The TriCinch System reproduces the Kay procedure by cinching at the anteroposterior commissure, thus reducing septolateral dimensions and preserving native anatomy. An 18F steerable delivery system is advanced through a 24F femoral vein introducer sheath into the right atrium. The device consists of a corkscrew anchor usually fixed at anteroposterior commissure. Once implanted, the corkscrew is connected to a nitinol stent delivered in the inferior vena cava using an adjustable Dacron band. Tension can be modulated while checking the effective reduction in the septolateral diameter and the impact on the TR. Implantation is completed with the deployment of the stent in the inferior vena cava. The procedure can be easily performed both under general sedation using transesophageal echocardiography or under conscious sedation with both fluoroscopy and intracardiac echocardiography. The Percutaneous Treatment of Tricuspid Valve Regurgitation with the TriCinch System (PREVENT) (NCT02098200) is an ongoing trial involving patients with severe FTR. Data report a successful procedure in 18 patients (85%) patients with a significant acute reduction of TR obtained in 94% of implanted patients. Two procedures were aborted, however, for hemopericardium; in 4 cases, a late anchor detachment was reported without any serious adverse event. The 6-month clinical follow-up was available for only 4 patients without mention of echocardiographic performance; data on the long-term efficacy of the device in terms of residual TR are needed. A second-generation device with an intrapericardial anchor to replace the annular anchor is being developed.

Trialign

The Trialign percutaneous tricuspid valve annuloplasty system consists of an articulating 8F wire catheter inserted through the jugular vein, a pledget catheter, and a plication lock device. The Trialign replicates the Kay surgical technique: 2 pledgets are fixed at the anteroposterior and septoposterior commissure and then sutured together using the dedicated plication lock device, thus plicating the posterior leaflet. In cases of suboptimal results, a second pair of pledgets can be implanted to obtain a consistent reduction in annular dimensions.[18] The safety and acute results of the device has been evaluated in the SCOUT I (Percutaneous Tricuspid Valve Annuloplasty

System for Symptomatic Chronic Functional Tricuspid Regurgitation), a study on 15 patients that demonstrated an acute implant success in all cases with 1 patient requiring RCA stenting. The investigators report a 30-day technical success rate of 80%, with 3 single-pledget annular detachments without any need of reintervention. The device implant significantly reduced the tricuspid annulus, effective regurgitant orifice area (EROA), and left ventricular stroke volume. In the intention-to-treat cohort, a significant improvement in New York Heart Association (NYHA) functional class ($\geq$1 class; P = .001), Minnesota Living with heart Failure Questionnaire (47.4 $\pm$ 17.6–20.9 $\pm$ 14.8; P<.001), and 6-minute walking test (245.2 $\pm$ 110.1–298.0 m $\pm$ 107.6 m; P = .008) was observed.[19] The multicenter experience on 14 patients treated for compassionate use reported a 42% of reduction in the vena contracta diameter and a significant reduction of annular area and annular diameters.[20] The ongoing SCOUT II trial has been initiated to support CE mark approval in Europe. The study is a nonrandomized, open-label clinical study recruiting 30 patients with evidence of FTR secondary to annular dilation.

SUMMARY

Percutaneous tricuspid valve annuloplasty represents a new a new therapeutic alternative for FTR. As the new era of the tricuspid valve is just beginning, preliminary data from the first feasibility trials should be considered because studies have to address safety and feasibility rather than efficacy. In the future, annuloplasty devices need to be evaluated in patients with less advanced right-sided heart failure without severe valvular remodeling in whom it is more likely to achieve better acute and long-term clinical results. The current ongoing studies (SCOUT II and TRI-REPAIR) represent an important step forward in the knowledge of percutaneous tricuspid annuloplasty and should be able to demonstrate excellent safety and at least moderate efficacy of these devices for the treatment of FTR. As a result, new percutaneous solutions could become commercially available for patients suffering from severe TR and address this important unmet clinical need.

REFERENCES

1. Mangieri A, Montalto C, Pagnesi M, et al. Mechanism and implications of the tricuspid regurgitation: from the pathophysiology to the current and future therapeutic options. Circ Cardiovasc Interv 2017;10(7) [pii: e005043].

2. Navia JL, Brozzi NA, Klein AL, et al. Moderate tricuspid regurgitation with left-sided degenerative heart valve disease: to repair or not to repair? Ann Thorac Surg 2012;93(1):59–67.

3. Rodés-Cabau J, Hahn RT, Latib A, et al. Transcatheter therapies for treating tricuspid regurgitation. J Am Coll Cardiol 2016;67(15):1829–45.

4. Taramasso M, Pozzoli A, Guidotti A, et al. Percutaneous tricuspid valve therapies: the new frontier. Eur Heart J 2017;38(9):639–47.

5. Rogers JH, Bolling SF. The tricuspid valve: current perspective and evolving management of tricuspid regurgitation. Circulation 2009;119(20):2718–25.

6. Taramasso M, Vanermen H, Maisano F, et al. The growing clinical importance of secondary tricuspid regurgitation. J Am Coll Cardiol 2012;59(8):703–10.

7. Antunes MJ, Barlow JB. Management of tricuspid valve regurgitation. Heart 2007;93(2):271–6.

8. Vahanian A, Alfieri O, Andreotti F, et al, ESC Committee for Practice Guidelines (CPG), Joint Task Force on the Management of Valvular Heart Disease of the European Society of Cardiology (ESC), European Association for Cardio-Thoracic Surgery (EACTS). Guidelines on the management of valvular heart disease (version 2012): the Joint Task Force on the Management of Valvular Heart Disease of the European Society of Cardiology (ESC) and the European Association for Cardio-Thoracic Surgery (EACTS). Eur J Cardiothorac Surg 2012;42(4):S1–44.

9. Latib A, Mangieri A. Transcatheter tricuspid valve repair: new valve, new opportunities, new challenges. J Am Coll Cardiol 2017;69(14):1807–10.

10. Van Rosendael PJ, Delgado V, Bax JJ. The tricuspid valve and the right heart: anatomical, pathological and imaging specifications. EuroIntervention 2015;11(Suppl W):W123–7.

11. Ancona F, Stella S, Taramasso M, et al. Multimodality imaging of the tricuspid valve with implication for percutaneous repair approaches. Heart 2017;103(14):1073–81.

12. Van Rosendael PJ, Kamperidis V, Kong WK, et al. Computed tomography for planning transcatheter tricuspid valve therapy. Eur Heart J 2017;38(9):665–74.

13. Hahn RT, Meduri CU, Davidson CJ, et al. Cardioband, a transcatheter surgical-like direct mitral valve annuloplasty system: early results of the feasibility trial. Eur Heart J 2016;37:817–25.

14. Latib A, Agricola E, Pozzoli A, et al. First-in-Man implantation of a tricuspid annular remodeling device for functional tricuspid regurgitation. JACC Cardiovasc Interv 2015;8(13):e211–4.

15. Taramasso M. Tricuspid repair with cardioband. Paper presented at: Transcatheter Cardiovascular

Therapeutics. Washington, DC, October 29, 2016.

16. Rogers JH. Millipede: evolution of the concept. Paper presented at: Transcatheter Valve Therepies. Chicago (IL), June 17, 2016.

17. Rogers T, Lederman RJ. Trans-atrial intra-pericardial tricuspid annuloplasty (TRAIPTA). Paper presented at: Transcatheter Cardiovascular Therapeutics. Chicago (IL), October 29, 2016.

18. Schofer J, Bijuklic K, Tiburtius C, et al. First-in-human transcatheter tricuspid valve repair in a patient with severely regurgitant tricuspid valve. J Am Coll Cardiol 2015;65(12):1190–5.

19. Hahn RT, Meduri CU, Davidson CJ, et al. Early feasibility study of a transcatheter tricuspid valve annuloplasty: SCOUT trial 30- day results. J Am Coll Cardiol 2017;69:1795–806.

20. Yzeiraj E. Early experience with the trialign system for transcatheter tricuspid valve repair: a multicenter experience. Paper presented at: Transcatheter Cardiovascular Therapeutics. Washington, DC, October 29, 2016.

Tricuspid Clip
Step-by-Step and Clinical Data

Gilbert H.L. Tang, MD, MSc, MBA

KEYWORDS

- Tricuspid regurgitation • MitraClip • Pacemaker lead

KEY POINTS

- Significant tricuspid regurgitation (TR) without treatment carries a dismal prognosis.
- Transcatheter tricuspid repair with the MitraClip system is safe.
- Patient screening using both transthoracic and transesophageal echocardiography is critical to assess procedural feasibility and extent of TR reduction.
- Integrating echocardiographic and fluoroscopic imaging simplifies device orientation and facilitates leaflet grasping and procedural success.
- The dedicated TriClip system and clips with longer grip arms may further improve ease of transcatheter tricuspid repair and clinical outcomes.

INTRODUCTION

Significant tricuspid regurgitation (TR) is a serious problem with few effective treatment options. Most cases are secondary to mitral regurgitation (MR) but a segment of the patient population may have primary TR caused by degenerative or congenital disease.[1,2] Untreated patients develop progressive right ventricular volume overload and dilatation, right heart failure, and the sequelae of peripheral edema and chronic liver congestion. Pacemaker or automatic implantable cardioverter defibrillator (AICD) lead-associated TR is common and these patients have higher mortality and morbidity than those without a right ventricular (RV) lead.[3,4] Prognosis in patients with untreated TR remains poor and surgery to repair or replace the tricuspid valve (TV) carries significant mortality and morbidity.[1,2] Current guidelines recommend a more aggressive approach in surgical repair of significant TR but many patients remain on medical therapy only.[1,2]

Transcatheter tricuspid repair with MitraClip has recently been shown to improve cardiac output in an ex-vivo model.[5] The system, designed for transcatheter mitral repair, recently emerged as a feasible treatment options in patients with significant TR deemed high risk for surgery.[6–21] More than 300 procedures have been performed worldwide and preliminary results are promising.[20,21] This article summarizes the step-by-step approach to TV repair with the MitraClip system and discusses currently available data.

PREPROCEDURAL SCREENING
Echocardiography

High-quality echocardiographic imaging is critical to determine the feasibility of tricuspid repair with the MitraClip system. Recent guidelines and reviews have been written on comprehensive echocardiographic evaluation of the TV.[22,23] Transthoracic echocardiography (TTE) is the initial study to acquire to determine TR severity and anatomy (Table 1), followed by transesophageal echocardiography (TEE) to determine whether the tricuspid anatomy, location, and severity of the TR jet, and TEE views will be adequate for leaflet grasping (Table 2). In patients with an RV lead, it is important to ensure that the lead will not cause excessive acoustic shadowing and its position will not

---

Conflicts of Interest: Dr G.H.L. Tang is a physician consultant for Abbott Structural Heart.
Department of Cardiovascular Surgery, Mount Sinai Health System, 1190 Fifth Avenue, GP2W, Box 1028, New York, NY 10029, USA
E-mail address: gilbert.tang@mountsinai.org

Intervent Cardiol Clin 7 (2018) 37–45
https://doi.org/10.1016/j.iccl.2017.09.001

Table 1
Transthoracic echocardiographic views and parameters to evaluate tricuspid valve repair with MitraClip system

I. Parasternal long-axis view	• LVOT with and without color Doppler (include zoomed view) • AV with and without zoomed view
II. Parasternal inflow view of TV	• TV with and without color Doppler CW • Doppler aligned with TR jet PW Doppler at level of TV annulus • PW Doppler at level of TV leaflet tips • PISA of TR jet
III. Parasternal outflow view of PV	• PV with and without color • Doppler PW of PV • CW of PV
IV. Parasternal short-axis view	• 2D RV (base, mid-RV, apex levels) • 2D TV (leaflet level: anterior, posterior, and septal), tips of TV leaflets • Color Doppler of TV over TV orifice
V. Basal parasternal short-axis view (level of AV)	• PV with and without color • Doppler TV with and without color Doppler • Pulsed Doppler of pulmonary flow at PV level If image well aligned: • CW Doppler aligned with TR jet PW Doppler at level of TV annulus • PW Doppler at level of TV leaflet tips • PISA TR jet
VI. Apical 4-chamber view	• 2D TV with and without color Doppler • CW Doppler of TR jet • PW Doppler at level of TV annulus • PW Doppler at level of TV leaflet tips PISA TR jet • Tissue Doppler of TV annulus • 2D RA with TV in middle of sector (include zoomed view) • RV (basal and annulus levels) (include zoomed view)
VII. Subcostal view	• IVC with and without a sniff • Color Doppler of IVC and hepatic vein • Pulsed Doppler of hepatic vein (forward and reversed flow) If image well aligned: • CW Doppler aligned with TR jet • PW Doppler at level of TV annulus • PW Doppler at level of TV leaflet tips • PISA TR jet
VIII. M mode	• LV/RV below tips of MV/TV leaflets

Abbreviations: AV, aortic valve; CW, continuous wave; 2D, two-dimensional; IVC, inferior vena cava; LV, left ventricle; LVOT, left ventricular outflow tract; PISA, proximal isovelocity surface area; PV, pulmonic valve; PW, pulse wave; RA, right atrium; RV, right ventricle; TR, tricuspid regurgitation; TV, tricuspid valve.

interfere with the clip delivery system (CDS) positioning and leaflet grasping. RV lead extraction may be an option in patients who are not pacer dependent and require an AICD.[19] Patients who are pacer dependent may instead have a coronary sinus or left ventricular lead implanted, or placement of a leadless pacemaker.[19] Those who need the benefit of an AICD may benefit from a subcutaneous device instead.

The 3 critical TEE views to determine the anatomy of the TR jet and feasibility of repair with MitraClip are:

1. Four-chamber view to visualize septal and anterior/posterior leaflets
2. TV inflow-outflow view (equivalent to bicommissural view of mitral valve [MV]) with X-plane to visualize septal and anterior/posterior leaflets for leaflet grasping
3. Transgastric basal short-axis view to visualize all 3 leaflets, and to determine TR jet location and width, and septal leaflet mobility

Three-dimensional (3D) TEE is helpful to visualize the 3 leaflets and device positioning relative to various commissures and leaflets.

Table 2
Transesophageal echocardiographic views and parameters to evaluate tricuspid valve repair with MitraClip system

I. Simultaneous multiplane view	• TV modified bicaval view as primary with and without color Doppler • TV inflow-outflow view as primary with and without color Doppler • TV 4-chamber view as primary with and without color • Doppler
II. ME modified bicaval view (TV commissural view)	• CW Doppler of TR jet PW of TV • TV inflow (annulus level) • TV tips
III. ME inflow-outflow view	• CW Doppler of TR jet PW of TV • TV inflow (annulus level) TV tips • 3D of RV
IV. 4-Chamber view (with deep esophageal 4-chamber view)	• CW Doppler of TR jet PW of TV • TV inflow (annulus level) TV tips • 3D of RV
V. 3D TV acquisition (recommended)	• TV at midesophageal angles 0°, 30°, and 60°, and deep gastric view angles 0° and 90° and with and without color Doppler
VI. Midesophageal 5-chamber view	• TV with and without color Doppler
VII. Midesophageal 4-chamber view	• TV with and without color Doppler
VIII. Midesophageal inflow-outflow view	• RVOT • 2D PV with and without color Doppler
IX. Midesophageal AV long-axis view	• RVOT • 2D PV with and without color Doppler
X. Midesophageal short-axis view	• RVOT • 2D PV with and without color Doppler
XI. Transgastric basal short-axis view	• TV with and without color Doppler
XII. Transgastric RV basal view	• TV with and without color Doppler
XIII. Transgastric RV inflow-outflow view	• TV with and without color Doppler
XIV. Deep gastric view	• PW the RVOT
XV. Ventricular view	• Focused views of RV

Abbreviations: 3D, three-dimensional; ME, midesophageal; RVOT, right ventricular outflow tract.

However, given that the TV leaflets are thinner than mitral leaflets, there may be acoustic drop-off on 3D and it may not be possible to visualize the leaflets completely. Another useful feature of 3D TEE is the localization of the RV lead across the TV to determine its location and the feasibility of repair with MitraClip given potential interference.

Cardiac Catheterization

Patients being considered for tricuspid repair with MitraClip should undergo left and right heart cardiac catheterization. Patients in active heart failure should be optimized medically to assess whether the TR severity may improve. Those with significant MR should be addressed first before TV repair. Concomitant MV and TV repair with Mitra-Clip can be performed but the procedural time is

significantly prolonged, and in certain patients TR improves after MitraClip repair, without the need to intervene on the TR.[24,25] Patients with moderate to severe pulmonary hypertension (systolic pulmonary arterial pressure >60 mm Hg) or significant RV dysfunction may not benefit from transcatheter TV repair, and are currently excluded from the TRILUMINATE (Trial to Evaluate Treatment with Abbott Transcatheter Clip Repair System in Patients with Moderate or Greater Tricuspid Regurgitation) trial (Clinicaltrials.gov identifier: NCT03227757).

Computed Tomography

The inferior vena caval anatomy should be evaluated before TV repair with MitraClip. A non-contrast computed tomography of the chest, abdomen, and pelvis is performed to identify any tortuosity or congenital anomaly making the TV repair with MitraClip potentially challenging or not feasible.

PROCEDURE STEP BY STEP

The transjugular approach to MitraClip TV repair has been reported but has largely been abandoned because of the length of the steerable guide catheter (SGC) and operator positioning.[7,12] Two techniques to perform MitraClip TV repair via the transfemoral approach have been described.[8,9,15,19] The classic technique refers to the CDS being inserted in the standard fashion into the SGC,[7,8] whereas the miskey technique refers to the CDS rotated counterclockwise by 90° before inserting into the SGC.[14,18] The miskey offers the potential advantage of the CDS straddling across the SGC tip enabling more versatile knob movements of the MitraClip system. The remainder of this article focuses on TV repair with MitraClip using the miskey technique.

TEE with 3D capability is essential to perform TV repair with MitraClip safely. TTE and intracardiac echocardiography (ICE) may serve as adjuncts when TEE images are limited, particularly during leaflet grasping to ensure adequate leaflet insertion.[17,18]

Access

- Percutaneous right femoral venous access is performed similar to the MitraClip procedure. A small stab incision with a #11 blade at the access site facilitates subsequent SGC insertion.
- One to 2 ProGlide sutures (Abbott Vascular, Santa Clara, CA) may be deployed at the beginning to facilitate subsequent percutaneous closure.
- Intravenous heparin is administered to a target activated clotting time greater than 300 seconds.
- Before SGC insertion, the authors place a #1 monofilament suture in a horizontal mattress fashion around the access site with a snare placed. Snaring of the suture facilitates external manual compression if access site hemostasis cannot be achieved, and the suture is secured at the end of the procedure for hemostasis. The suture is removed in postprocedural day 1.
- After placing a 7-French (F) sheath, a stiff guidewire can be advanced to the superior vena cava and the sheath can be exchanged with the SGC after serial dilation with 14-F then 18-F dilators.

Steerable Guide Catheter and Clip Delivery System Insertion

- The SGC is inserted in the standard fashion as a MitraClip procedure, with the initial plus/minus (+/−) knob turned 180° to the minus (−) direction to straighten the tip.
- Afterward, return the plus/minus (+/−) knob to neutral position and turn the SGC 180° with the plus/minus (+/−) knob facing downward (**Fig. 1A,B**).
- Insert the CDS with the blue line rotated 90° counterclockwise (miskey) and exit the SGC straddled (**Fig. 1C**).

Clip Steering to the Tricuspid Valve

- Under TEE and fluoroscopic guidance, at a left anterior oblique (LAO) projection, turn the SGC clockwise while turning the A knob slowly to steer the clip toward the TV (**Fig. 1D; Fig. 2A–D**).
- At LAO projection the clip should be swinging leftward down toward the TV along the right atrial wall. Swinging the clip rightward would be toward the interatrial septum and may impede the steering down toward the TV (see **Fig. 2A,B**).
- Once the clip is visualized by TEE to be above the TV, rotate the C-arm to right anterior oblique (RAO) projection to visualize the longitudinal view of the TV (**Fig. 2E,F**). This is the fluoroscopic grasping view.

Clip Orientation and Crossing the Tricuspid Valve

- The target anatomy and location (eg, anterior/septal leaflet) of the MitraClip implantation should be determined before the procedure (**Fig. 3A**). With the clip above the TV annulus, use the LAO projection on fluoroscopy in combination with 3D TEE to orient the clip to suit the target location (**Fig. 3B**).
- Once oriented, close the clip to 60° to avoid entanglement with the TV leaflets or RV lead, and advance the clip slowly on RAO projection into the RV just below the TV. Beware of RV injury if the CDS is advanced too deep into the RV (**Fig. 3C**).

Clip Positioning and Leaflet Grasping

- Open the clip and fine tune the orientation at LAO projection and using the transgastric short-axis view on TEE.

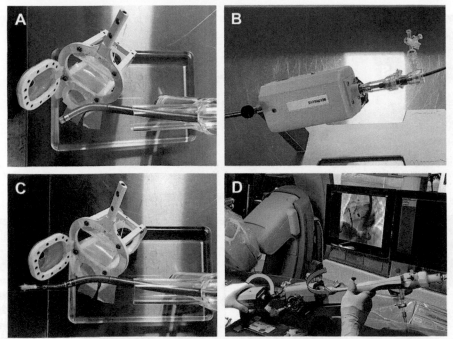

Fig. 1. (*A*) Anterior-posterior view of the SGC positioned in the right atrium, relative to the TV, in a demonstration model. (*B*) After SGC insertion, it is turned 180° with the (+/−) knob facing downward. (*C*) Inserting the CDS using the miskey technique allows the CDS to straddle across the tip of SGC, with the anterior-posterior view showing that the MitraClip is positioned at the superior vena cava/right atrial junction. (*D*) Intraprocedural view of the MitraClip system steering from the right atrium to the TV annulus.

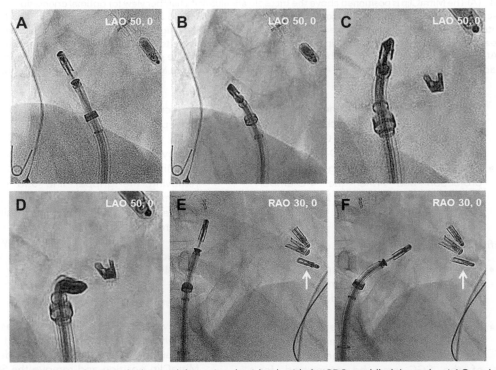

Fig. 2. (*A–D*) Turning the SGC clockwise while turning the A knob with the CDS straddled showed on LAO projection that the MitraClip is steered away from the interatrial septum (seen by the Amplatzer device) toward the TV. The position of the prior MitraClip placed at the TV can serve as a reference. (*E, F*). Right anterior oblique (RAO) projection shows the steering of the MitraClip toward the TV. Note the existing MitraClip already placed at the TV (*white arrows*).

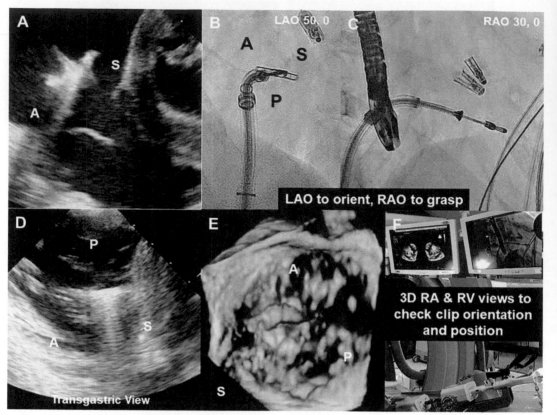

Fig. 3. (*A*) The MitraClip is positioned above the tricuspid annulus at 4-chamber view for optimal orientation. (*B*) LAO projection corresponds with the approximate orientation of the MitraClip targeted toward the anterior and septal leaflets. (*C*) Use the RAO projection to advance the MitraClip toward the right ventricle. (*D*) Deep transgastric basal short-axis view can visualize the MitraClip orientation and position relative to the leaflets, which can be corroborated on LAO projection. (*E*, *F*) 3D TEE using both RA and RV views can optimize positioning and orientation of the Mitra-Clip across anterior and septal leaflets. A, anterior; P, posterior; RA, right atrium; RV, right ventricle; S, septal.

Maneuver the clip toward the target area under these 2 views, then change to the grasping view on TEE. Confirm clip position on 3D TEE (**Fig. 3D–F**).

- Grasp the leaflets using the RAO projection and either the 4-chamber view or RV inflow-outflow X-plane view on TEE (**Fig. 4A,B**).

Confirming leaflet insertion and clip release

- Once the leaflets are grasped, confirm leaflet insertion by using multiple views and on 3D TEE. Assess degree of TR reduction.
- If a central venous catheter is present, measure the change in central venous pressure. Alternatively, the side port of the SGC may be connected for continuous hemodynamic monitoring of right atrial pressure and V wave. Significant TR reduction should result in

a decrease in central venous or right atrial pressure.

- Once leaflet insertion is confirmed, deploy the clip in the same fashion as the MitraClip. Pay special attention when removing the gripper line and do so extremely slowly because the sharp needle of the CDS can more easily go forward toward the TV and clip, unlike mitral repair. Assess clip anatomy and TR reduction using multiple TEE views (**Fig. 4C–E**).

Delivery system removal and closure

- Remove the CDS in a similar fashion. Straighten the SGC and turn back to the regular orientation similar to the default MitraClip position and remove the SGC.
- Perform standard femoral venous closure with ProGlide sutures and confirm hemostasis.

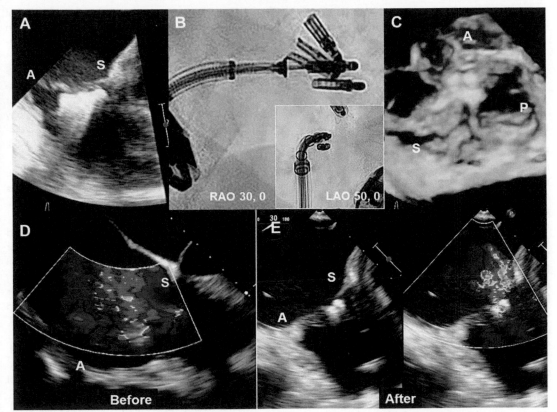

Fig. 4. (A) Ensure on TEE that both leaflets are visible during grasping. (B) Use RAO projection for leaflet grasping and LAO projection to determine relative orientation and position of the MitraClip during grasping, to avoid interaction with prior clip placed at the TV. (C) 3D TEE shows a tissue bridge across the anterior and septal leaflets confirming adequate leaflet insertion without detachment. (D) TEE showing torrential TR before MitraClip procedure. (E) Residual moderate TR after 2 MitraClips placed at anterior and septal leaflets.

PRESENCE OF A RIGHT VENTRICULAR LEAD

An RV lead is not a contraindication to performing TV repair with MitraClip. However, the lead must not be overly echogenic and negatively affect imaging quality on TEE. The lead should not be in a position to interfere with the CDS movement and ideally should not be tethered to the septal leaflet preventing adequate leaflet grasping. Lead extraction before transcatheter TV repair may make the procedure easier that may otherwise preclude the patient from receiving the therapy.[19]

TROUBLESHOOTING AND TIPS

TV repair with MitraClip is safe and complications are rare. However, a few technical challenges unique to the tricuspid anatomy deserve attention:

- The tricuspid leaflets are thin and fragile, especially in secondary TR. Ensure good leaflet insertion before lowering the grippers and closing the clip arms because repeat leaflet grasping may risk leaflet tearing and worsening TR.
- Ensure that the clip arms are optimally aligned with the grasping leaflets. Because the TV leaflets are thinner, if the alignment is not perpendicular to the grasp plane, after the clip is deployed the clip may spin and distort the TV leaflets, causing more TR.
- Avoid advancing the CDS too deep into the RV because the RV cavity is usually smaller than the left ventricle.
- Entanglement with the TV leaflets and chords can be more likely given the smaller septal leaflet and chordal attachments to the septum. Slow, purposeful movements of the CDS are key to avoiding chordal or leaflet laceration.
- Advance the clip partly closed at the center of the TV orifice to minimize the risk of leaflet and chordal interaction.

- Applying pressure on the anterior chest at the distal sternum (similar to performing cardiopulmonary resuscitation) may help reduce RV and TV annular dimensions to improve leaflet grasping. This technique has been anecdotally reported but results have not been consistent.

CLINICAL EVIDENCE

Residual significant TR, even after MitraClip mitral repair, leads to poorer clinical outcomes.[24,25] TR associated with an RV lead is common and may benefit from lead extraction to improve the TR or to facilitate MitraClip repair.[4,19] Tricuspid repair with the MitraClip system has had excellent safety outcomes in more than 100 reported patients.[6–21] In the TriValve Registry, 58 of 106 patients underwent MitraClip repair.[20] Nickenig and colleagues[16] reported the largest series of 64 consecutive patients who underwent either an isolated TV or combined TV and MV MitraClip procedure.[16] Procedural success was 97% and 91% of patients had at least 1 grade TR reduction. No major complications occurred and most patients had New York Heart Association class improvement at discharge and increased 6-minute walk test at 30 days. MitraClip has also been successfully used in TV repair for degenerative and congenital TR.[9–13] The TRILUMINATE is a 25-center, 75-patient global feasibility trial to perform tricuspid repair with the TriClip system in patients with symptomatic moderate or greater TR. Enrollment has begun and the trial should be completed by early 2018.

SUMMARY

Transcatheter TV repair with the MitraClip system is a safe and promising treatment option in patients with symptomatic significant TR deemed high risk for surgery. Although the presence of a pacemaker/AICD lead is not a contraindication, careful patient screening using TTE and TEE is critical to determine procedural feasibility and potential success. Combining echocardiographic and fluoroscopic guidance simplifies the procedure, facilitates leaflet grasping and deployment, and avoids potential complications. Ongoing optimal medical therapy remains necessary to sustain the benefits of transcatheter tricuspid repair. The clinical efficacy of the dedicated TriClip system will be evaluated in the TRILUMINATE trial.

REFERENCES

1. Nishimura RA, Otto CM, Bonow RO, et al. 2014 AHA/ACC guideline for the management of patients with valvular heart disease: a report of the American College of Cardiology/American Heart Association Task Force on Practice Guidelines. J Thorac Cardiovasc Surg 2014;148:e1–132.
2. Baumgartner H, Falk V, Bax JJ, et al. 2017 ESC/EACTS guidelines for the management of valvular heart disease: The Task force for the management of valvular heart disease of the European Society of Cardiology (ESC) and the European Association for Cardio-Thoracic Surgery (EACTS). Eur Heart J 2017;1–53. https://doi.org/10.1093/eurheartj/ehx391.
3. Delling FN, Hassan ZK, Piatkowski G, et al. Tricuspid regurgitation and mortality in patients with transvenous permanent pacemaker leads. Am J Cardiol 2016;117:988–92.
4. Chang JD, Manning WJ, Ebrille E, et al. Tricuspid valve dysfunction following pacemaker or cardioverter-defibrillator implantation. J Am Coll Cardiol 2017;69:2331–41.
5. Vismara R, Gelpi G, Prabhu S, et al. Transcatheter edge-to-edge treatment of functional tricuspid regurgitation in an ex vivo pulsatile heart model. J Am Coll Cardiol 2016;68:1024–33.
6. Schofer J, Tiburtius C, Hammerstingl C, et al. Transfemoral tricuspid valve repair using a percutaneous mitral valve repair system. J Am Coll Cardiol 2016;67:889–90.
7. Hammerstingl C, Schueler R, Malasa M, et al. Transcatheter treatment of severe tricuspid regurgitation with the MitraClip system. Eur Heart J 2016;37:849–53.
8. Wengenmayer T, Zehender M, Bothe W, et al. First transfemoral percutaneous edge-to-edge repair of the tricuspid valve using the MitraClip system. EuroIntervention 2016;11:1541–4.
9. Braun D, Nabauer M, Massberg S, et al. Transcatheter repair of primary tricuspid valve regurgitation using the MitraClip system. JACC Cardiovasc Interv 2016;9:e153–4.
10. Lesevic H, Frangieh AH, Kasel AM, et al. Successful percutaneous edge-to-edge repair in degenerative tricuspid valve regurgitation using the MitraClip system. Eur Heart J 2017;38:691.
11. Picard F, Tadros VX, Asgar AW. From tricuspid to double orifice morphology: percutaneous tricuspid regurgitation repair with the MitraClip device in congenitally corrected-transposition of great arteries. Catheter Cardiovasc Interv 2016. https://doi.org/10.1002/ccd.26834.
12. Latib A, Mangieri A, Agricola E, et al. Percutaneous bicuspidalization of the tricuspid valve using the MitraClip system. Int J Cardiovasc Imaging 2017;33:227–8.
13. Fam NP, Connelly KA, Hammerstingl C, et al. Transcatheter tricuspid repair with MitraClip for severe primary tricuspid regurgitation. J Invasive Cardiol 2016;28:E223–4.

14. Gafoor S, Petrescu OM, Lehr EJ, et al. Percutaneous tricuspid valve regurgitation repair with the MitraClip device using an edge-to-edge bicuspidization technique. J Invasive Cardiol 2017;29:E30–6.

15. Braun D, Nabauer M, Orban M, et al. Transcatheter treatment of severe tricuspid regurgitation using the edge-to-edge repair technique. EuroIntervention 2017;12:e1837–44.

16. Nickenig G, Kowalski M, Hausleiter J, et al. Transcatheter treatment of severe tricuspid regurgitation with the edge-to-edge MitraClip technique. Circulation 2017;135:1802–14.

17. Avenatti E, Barker CM, Little SH. Tricuspid regurgitation repair with a MitraClip device: the pivotal role of 3D transoesophageal echocardiography. Eur Heart J Cardiovasc Imaging 2017;18:380.

18. Pozzoli A, Taramasso M, Zuber M, et al. Transcatheter tricuspid valve repair with MitraClip system using intracardiac echocardiography: proof of concept. EuroIntervention 2017. https://doi.org/10.4244/EIJ-D-17-00360 [pii:EIJ-D-17-00360].

19. Tang GH, Kaple R, Cohen M, et al. First percutaneous Micra leadless pacemaker implantation and tricuspid valve repair with MitraClip NT for lead-associated severe tricuspid regurgitation. EuroIntervention 2017;12:e1845–8.

20. Regazzoli D, Ielasi A, Lanzillo G, et al. Sustained reduction of tricuspid regurgitation after percutaneous repair with the MitraClip system in a patient with a dual chamber pacemaker. JACC Cardiovasc Interv 2017;10:e147–9.

21. Taramasso M, Hahn RT, Alessandrini H, et al. International multicenter transcatheter tricuspid valve therapies (TriValve) registry: which patients are undergoing transcatheter tricuspid repair? JACC Cardiovasc Interv 2017;10(19):1982–90.

22. Hahn RT, Abraham T, Adams MS, et al. Guidelines for performing a comprehensive transesophageal echocardiographic examination: recommendations from the American Society of Echocardiography and the Society of Cardiovascular Anesthesiologists. J Am Soc Echocardiogr 2013;26:921–64.

23. Hahn RT. State-of-the-art review of echocardiographic imaging in the evaluation and treatment of functional tricuspid regurgitation. Circ Cardiovasc Imaging 2016;9 [pii:e005332].

24. Toyama K, Ayabe K, Kar S, et al. Postprocedural changes of tricuspid regurgitation after MitraClip therapy for mitral regurgitation. Am J Cardiol 2017;120(5):857–61.

25. Kalbacher D, Schäfer U, von Bardeleben RS, et al. Impact of tricuspid valve regurgitation in surgical high-risk patients undergoing MitraClip implantation: results from the TRAMI registry. EuroIntervention 2017;12:e1809–16.

The FORMA Repair System

Rishi Puri, MBBS, PhD, Josep Rodés-Cabau, MD*

KEYWORDS

- Tricuspid regurgitation • Tricuspid annular dilatation • FORMA device
- Percutaneous tricuspid valve repair

KEY POINTS

- Functional tricuspid insufficiency invariably results from right ventricular and subsequent tricuspid annular dilatation leading to tricuspid leaflet malcoaptation or noncoaptation. The FORMA Repair System has been designed to reduce the regurgitant orifice area by providing a surface for valve leaflet coaptation.
- The initial human experience in elderly, high-surgical-risk, inoperable patients showed procedural safety, with 16 patients undergoing 1-year clinical follow-up.
- Clinical benefits seem to be evident early postprocedure, with noticeable improvements in functional capacity and right heart failure, maintained at 1 year in most cases.
- Only partial correction of tricuspid insufficiency is observed in most FORMA recipients on imaging, with ongoing challenges remaining regarding the classification of tricuspid insufficiency severity in the setting of in situ Spacer devices.
- Two large clinical registries are currently underway to further evaluate the safety and efficacy of the FORMA Repair System.

INTRODUCTION

Tricuspid regurgitation (TR), in most cases, arises from right ventricular (RV) dilatation, which in turn may be a result of numerous disorders involving either RV pressure or volume overload. These disorders may include left-sided heart disease with subsequent pulmonary arterial hypertension, precapillary pulmonary hypertension, or RV infarction with subsequent adverse RV remodeling. Thus, tricuspid valve (TV) annular dilatation represents the dominant mechanism of secondary, or functional TR.[1] Progressive tricuspid annular dilation occurs in its anteroposterior plane, corresponding with the free wall of the RV. Significant TR occurs when the anterior and posterior leaflets are pulled away from their coaptation point, resulting in jets of TR. Leaflet tethering develops during more advanced stages of RV dilatation and papillary muscle displacement. RV annular dilatation and TV leaflet malcoaptation thus serves as the chief pathologic substrate for the design and development of the FORMA Repair System (Edwards Lifesciences, Irvine, CA); a tricuspid Spacer designed to occupy the effective regurgitant orifice.

THE FORMA REPAIR SYSTEM
Device Concept and Design

The Edwards FORMA Tricuspid Valve Repair System represents a novel, fully percutaneous treatment option for patients with moderate-severe TR.[2] The chief design element involves placing a device to reduce the TR regurgitant orifice area, thereby providing a surface for valve native leaflet coaptation. The device consists of a Spacer and a rail, which is anchored within the right ventricular apex (Fig. 1). The Spacer passively expands via holes within the Spacer shaft. Position of the Spacer across the annulus can be confirmed with the guidance of TEE. In the advent of significant leaflet teth- ering/restriction resulting in a very

Disclosure: Dr J. Rodés-Cabau has received research grants from Edwards Lifesciences. Dr R. Puri has no disclosures.
Quebec Heart and Lung Institute, Laval University, 2725 Chemin Ste-Foy, Quebec City, QC G1V 4G5, Canada
* Corresponding author.
E-mail address: josep.rodes@criucpq.ulaval.ca

Intervent Cardiol Clin 7 (2018) 47–55
http://dx.doi.org/10.1016/j.iccl.2017.08.007

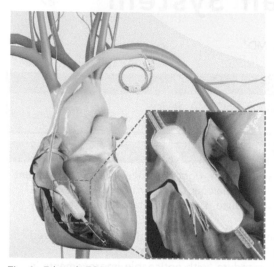

Fig. 1. Edwards FORMA Tricuspid Valve Repair System for the treatment of tricuspid regurgitation through a transcatheter approach. (*Courtesy of* Edwards Lifesciences Corporation, Inc, Irvine, CA; with permission.)

large regurgitant orifice, the Spacer can be adjusted in both the ventricular/atrial and superior/inferior directions in the annulus to attempt to further reduce the TR. The Spacer cannot be adjusted in the septal/lateral direction unless there is an attempt to re-anchor at a different location in the RV apex. There are currently two available coaptation diameter sizes (12-mm and 15-mm), with other diameter sizes under current development for clinical use. Overall Spacer length is 42-mm with two radiopaque markers to position the Spacer using fluoroscopy. The device is positioned such that the Spacer occupies the regurgitant space and is ultimately fixed proximally in the right ventricular myocardium. The fixation mechanism consists of a six-pronged nitinol anchor, designed to minimize the risk of perforation. The device may be removed percutaneously.

Patient Selection

Clinical indications currently include severe TR in the presence of symptomatic right heart failure deemed by the heart team to be at very high or prohibitive surgical risk. Patients with PPM leads can and have been successfully treated, however one needs to consider potential anatomic constraints that may obviate the placement of a Spacer device in these scenarios. Patients with prior TV surgery were excluded. Transthoracic and transesophageal echocardiography, along with computed tomography (CT), are essential for preprocedural patient selection and planning. Key issues involve assessing not only the severity and mechanism of TR, annular dimensions, and right ventricular geometry but also the status of

subclavian venous access to ensure an adequate size to facilitate the introducer sheath and device. Indeed there are certain general anatomic requirements to optimize Spacer placement and positioning. A prominent moderator band may/may not interfere. The CT is used as an important screening tool to assess the TV subvalvular apparatus, structures/anatomy that would preclude successful navigation, positioning and retrieval of the Spacer device.

The initial first-in-human clinical experience, comprising 7 patients across 2 centers, has been reported in detail.[3] Ongoing clinical experience has gradually evolved and, to date, 1-year clinical data are currently available in 15 patients across 3 centers in Canada and Switzerland.[4] These patients had severe symptomatic TR and were assessed by the respective institutional heart teams to be inoperable because of unacceptably high surgical risk. The Canadian patients were treated under a special access protocol approved by Health Canada, and the Swiss patients were treated under the conditions of the Compassionate Use Program of the Swiss Agency for Therapeutic products (Swissmedic). All patients provided informed consent for the procedures. Important exclusions included primary TR or prior tricuspid surgery. Patients with pacemakers or defibrillators were included after enrollment of the first 15 patients.

Procedural Imaging

Transthoracic echocardiography (TTE) and transesophageal echocardiography (TEE) were both performed preprocedure to estimate TR severity according to current clinical guidelines.[5,6] Intraprocedure, TEE guidance served to localize the implantation site and confirm correct anchoring of the device within the septal segment of the myocardium of the RV apex. Device positioning was optimized using continuous echocardiographic TR surveillance. In the setting of an RV pacemaker lead, TEE was used to exclude adhesion of the pacemaker lead to any of the valve leaflets.

All patients underwent electrocardiogram-synchronized multidetector cardiac CT. The recorded images were used to measure tricuspid annular dimension, midventricular diameter, and the distance from the TV annulus to the RV apex. In addition, the configuration of the subvalvular apparatus, including the position of the papillary muscles, the moderator band, and pacing leads, was assessed. The target anchoring site was selected based on a sagittal CT reconstruction perpendicular to the tricuspid annulus by drawing a perpendicular line linking the tricuspid plane with the RV septal free wall groove (**Fig. 2**) (Circle Cardiovascular Imaging, Calgary, Alberta). Based on this projection, a fluoroscopic angulation allowing perpendicular representation of the tricuspid annulus was defined.

Procedural Steps

Fluoroscopic guidance (**Fig. 3**) coupled with two-dimensional (2D) and three-dimensional (3D) TEE was used. Following left axillary venous access, a large-bore sheath (20 Fr for the 12-mm device, 24-Fr for the 15-mm device) is secured to accommodate the Spacer. Right ventriculography is performed to locate fluoroscopically the tricuspid annular plane and true right ventricular apex (see **Fig. 3A**). Ideally, the device should be positioned perpendicular to the valve plane to ensure optimal device coaptation. The anchor site is aimed at the RV wall perpendicular to the center of the annulus. A steerable delivery catheter is positioned within the RV for rail system delivery (see **Fig. 3B, C**). The Spacer is then tracked over the rail to the TV plane and placed in the best position to reduce TR, and this is assessed live

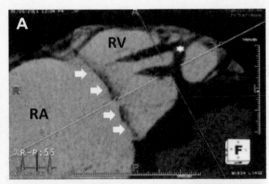

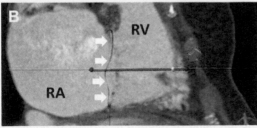

Fig. 2. Preprocedural contrast-enhanced CT imaging. (*A*) Anatomic structures of the right heart: right atrium (RA), RV, TV leaflets, and annular plane (*white arrows*) with a moderator band (*star*) (*B*) Sagittal reconstruction delineating the annular plane (*white arrows*) and the planned anchoring site (*yellow arrow*). (*From* Perlman G, Praz F, Puri R, et al. Transcatheter tricuspid valve repair with a new transcatheter coaptation system for the treatment of severe tricuspid regurgitation - one year clinical and echocardiographic results. JACC Cardiovasc Interv 2017; with permission.)

with echocardiography. The device is then locked proximally, and the excess rail length is coiled and placed within a subcutaneous pocket. If required, the entire device is fully retrievable during all stages of the procedure until sheath removal. The device could be removed weeks/months post insertion, not unlike an extrusion process for regular pacemaker leads, however.

FIRST-IN-HUMAN 1-YEAR RESULTS

Baseline Characteristics

Eighteen patients were treated with the FORMA system between February 2015 and July 2016. To date, all patients are being followed and 15 patients have undergone 1-year clinical follow-up.[4] Mean age was 76 ± 9.7 years, with a female preponderance (72%). As shown in **Table 1**, patients were high risk for surgery as estimated by a EuroSCORE II score of 9.1% ± 5.7%. Thirteen patients (72%) had a history of prior open heart surgery, most often left-sided valvular surgery (56%). Additional comorbidities included atrial fibrillation (AF) (89%) and severe pulmonary hypertension (33%).

At baseline, all patients reported fatigue and exertional dyspnea, with 67% having significant peripheral edema. Within the 12 months preceding the procedure, 10 patients (56%) required hospitalization for heart failure treatment, with the average daily dose of furosemide being 85 mg. New York Heart Association (NYHA) grade was 3 or more in 94% of participants and the average 6-minute walk test distance was 256 ± 103 m.

On baseline echocardiography, all but 1 patient presented with severe TR, with most showing vena contracta (VC) widths greater than 12 mm, which is compatible with effective regurgitant orifice areas (EROAs) greater than 120 mm^2 (torrential TR). All patients showed RV annular dilatation secondary to left-sided heart disease or pulmonary hypertension. Although RV dimensions were enlarged (mean annular diameter, 46 ± 6 mm), RV systolic function was preserved in most (83%) participants. The mean pulmonary artery systolic pressure was 43 ± 12 mm Hg.

Periprocedural and Hospital Course

Procedural characteristics are detailed in **Table 2**. Vascular access was achieved via the left subclavian or axillary veins in all cases, and surgical closure was performed in 72%. Mean skin-to-skin procedural time was 129 ± 36 minutes. Procedural success was achieved in 16 patients (89%). One patient's device dislocated into the

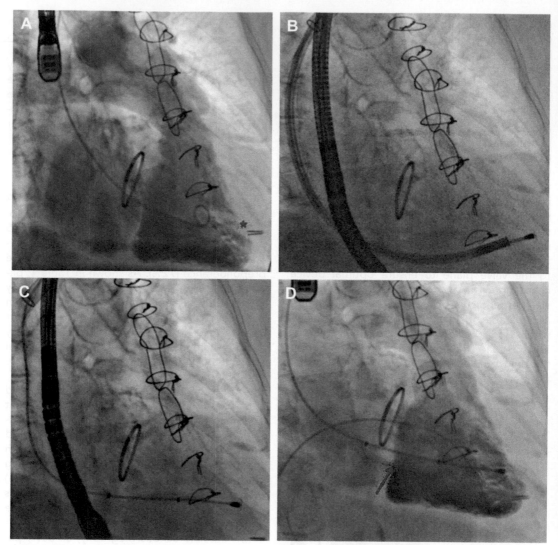

Fig. 3. Intraprocedural fluoroscopic/angiography. (*A*) Right ventriculography to locate the tricuspid annular plane and identify the ideal anchor location (*red asterisk*) on fluoroscopy. (*B*) Right ventricular anchoring via a steerable delivery catheter. (*C*) Device positioning in the valve plane. (*D*) Final right ventriculography showing the device in correct position (*red arrow*) and reduction of tricuspid regurgitation from baseline. (*From* Campelo-Parada F, Perlman G, Philippon F, et al. First-in-man experience of a novel transcatheter repair system for treating severe tricuspid regurgitation. J Am Coll Cardiol 2015;66(22):2478; with permission.)

right atrium a few hours following the intervention because of inadequate anchoring. A second patient experienced RV perforation during device positioning of the guiding catheter at the apex, necessitating emergent conversion to open surgical and subsequent, uneventful surgical tricuspid annuloplasty. There were no procedural deaths, myocardial infarctions, or pulmonary embolisms. One patient had a prolonged hospital course caused by pneumonia, mild access site bleeding, and mild acute kidney injury. Two patients had intraprocedural sustained ventricular ectopy that resolved with repositioning of the anchoring rail. Two other patients

had frequent premature ventricular beats that subsided within 24 hours under medical treatment (β-blockers). In 1 patient, paresthesia of the left hand developed as a result of an access site hematoma. Median hospital stay was 4 days (interquartile range, 2–5 days).

Clinical Outcomes at 1 Year
The periprocedural and 30-day outcomes in the first 7 patients across 2 centers, representing the first-in-human experience with this device, have been described in detail.[3] Since then, following further patient enrollment as well as the inclusion of a third center, the 1-year results of 15

Table 1 Baseline characteristics	
Characteristic	(n = 18)
Age (y)	76 ± 9.7
Female sex	13 (72)
Body mass index (kg/m^2)	27.2 ± 5.7
Serum creatinine level (µmol/L)	131 ± 74
Clinical Features of Heart Failure	
Exertional dyspnea	18 (100)
Lower extremity edema	12 (67)
Severe pulmonary hypertension[a]	6 (33)
B-type natriuretic peptide (pg/mL)	441 ± 432
N-terminal pro–B-type natriuretic peptide (pg/mL)	2812 ± 2798
Daily frusemide dose (mg[b])	85 ± 73
NYHA Functional Class	
II	1 (6)
III	14 (78)
IV	3 (17)
EuroSCORE II	9 ± 5.7
6-min walk test (m)	256 ± 103
Kansas City Cardiomyopathy Questionnaire	63.0 ± 20.4
Coexisting Conditions	
Hypertension	16 (89)
Diabetes	2 (11)
Creatinine clearance <30 mL/min (eGFR)	3 (17)
Atrial fibrillation	16 (89)
Coronary artery disease	10 (56)
Prior open heart surgery	13 (72)
Prior left-sided valve surgery	9 (50)
Aortic	4 (22)
Mitral	6 (33)
Stroke/TIA	2 (11)
COPD	5 (28)
Pacemaker/defibrillator	3 (17)

Values are mean ± SD or n (%).

Abbreviations: COPD, chronic obstructive pulmonary disease; eGFR, estimated glomerular filtration rate; NYHA, New York Heart Association; TIA, transient ischemic attack.

[a] Mean pulmonary artery pressure greater than 40 mm Hg or peak systolic pressure greater than 60 mm Hg, or specific medical treatment of pulmonary arterial hypertension.

[b] When patients received torsemide, a conversion ratio of 2:1 was used for calculating an equivalent dose of furosemide.

patients who have undergone 1-year clinical follow-up postprocedure are summarized here.[4]

1. Clinical events: there were no deaths, no surgical site or device infections, no pulmonary embolisms, and no significant arrhythmias requiring device or antiarrhythmic intervention (**Table 3**).
2. Functional status: significant improvement occurred by 30 days in patients with successful device implantation (n = 16), which was sustained at 1 year in the 14 patients who had functional status assessed at this time point. NYHA functional class improved in 12 out of 14 patients (86%) with a FORMA device in place at this time point. These functional improvements were translated into significant increases in the distance walked during 6 minutes and in the Kansas City Cardiomyopathy Questionnaire heart failure score (**Table 4**).
3. Heart failure surrogates: peripheral edema significantly improved compared with baseline, with 1 patient presenting with an edema score greater than 1 (ankle-level edema) compared with 13 patients with a score greater than 1 at baseline. Diuretic use also noticeably declined. N-terminal pro–B-type natriuretic peptide levels decreased in most patients (see **Table 4**).
4. Adverse device-related events: 1 patient, in the setting of subtherapeutic International Normalized Ratios, presented with device-related thrombosis (not apparent on a screening TTE 2 months earlier), which resolved following 2 months of therapeutic anticoagulation.

Echocardiographic Findings

At 30 days, 16 patients had evaluable echocardiographic follow-up, whereas, at 1 year, 13 patients had available echocardiography (2 patients had failed procedures, as described earlier, and 1 further patient had no available 1-year echocardiogram).[4] Thirty-day echocardiographic evaluation of TR showed a reduction in TR severity in all but 1 patient with a successfully implanted device. Residual moderate TR was observed in most cases. According to imaging guideline criteria, 5 patients still showed severe

From Perlman G, Praz F, Puri R, et al. Transcatheter tricuspid valve repair with a new transcatheter coaptation system for the treatment of severe tricuspid regurgitation - one year clinical and echocardiographic results. JACC Cardiovasc Interv 2017; with permission.

Table 2
Procedural characteristics

Characteristic	All Patients (n = 18)
Left subclavian vein access	17 (94)
Right subclavian vein access	1 (6)
Left-sided pacemaker present	2 (11)
Right-sided pacemaker present	1 (6)
FORMA Spacer Size Implanted	
15 mm	16 (89)
12 mm	1 (6)
Device oversizing (%)[a]	89 ± 100
Retrieval attempt/success	3 (17)/1 (6)
Venous closure	
Surgical	13 (72)
Perclose device	5 (28)
Procedure time, skin to skin (min)	129 ± 31
Fluoroscopy time (min)	24.7 ± 7.3
Contrast media (mL)	65 ± 29
Successful device implantation[b]	16 (89)
Dislocation of Spacer into right atrium	1 (6)
Conversion to surgery	1 (6)
Sustained ventricular arrhythmia	1 (6)
Mortality	0

Values are mean ± SD or n (%).
[a] Degree of oversizing was calculated as: [(device cross-sectional area − EROA)/EROA] × 100.
[b] A successful implantation of a FORMA Spacer in the TV resulting in an acute reduction of TR by at least 1 grade, with no need for surgical conversion or procedural death.
From Perlman G, Praz F, Puri R, et al. Transcatheter tricuspid valve repair with a new transcatheter coaptation system for the treatment of severe tricuspid regurgitation - one year clinical and echocardiographic results. JACC Cardiovasc Interv 2017; with permission.

Table 3
One-year clinical results

Outcome	1 y (n = 15)
Death	0
TIA	1 (7)
Myocardial infarction	0
Rehospitalization for heart failure	1 (7)
Access-related Bleeding	
Life threatening[a]	NA
Major[b]	NA
Minor	NA
Other bleeding events, minor GI	1 (7)
Vascular Complications	
Major	NA
Minor	NA
Hospital stay (median, IQR)	NA
Acute kidney injury ≥2	1 (7)
Sustained ventricular arrhythmia[c]	0
Pulmonary embolism	0
New pacemaker	0
Device thrombosis[d]	1 (7)
Infection[e]	4 (27)

Values are median (IQR) or n (%).
Abbreviations: GI, gastrointestinal; IQR, interquartile range; NA, not available.
[a] Tamponade from RV perforation that necessitated surgical repair.
[b] Pocket hematoma with nerve compression (paresthesia).
[c] Not occurring during the procedure.
[d] Occurred in a patient with nontherapeutic International Normalized Ratio levels, resolved with resumption of adequate anticoagulation.
[e] Three cases of pneumonia (twice in the same patient), 1 case of cholecystitis, and 1 case of leg cellulitis.
From Perlman G, Praz F, Puri R, et al. Transcatheter tricuspid valve repair with a new transcatheter coaptation system for the treatment of severe tricuspid regurgitation - one year clinical and echocardiographic results. JACC Cardiovasc Interv 2017; with permission.

TR, but there were no patients with very severe TR (Table 5). At 1 year of follow-up, 3 patients showed ongoing TR regression to mild to moderate severity. In contrast, 7 patients still showed residual severe TR. RV diameters significantly decreased compared with baseline measurements (mean diameter measured at the base of the RV, 49.9 ± 4.7 mm vs 55.1 ± 6.7 mm at baseline; $P = .02$). Echocardiographic evidence of reverse RV remodeling, defined as a sustained decrease in RV dimensions with concomitant evidence of significant reduction of TR, was found in 4 patients (28%).

Summary and Ongoing Future Perspectives

The totality of current clinical experience with the FORMA tricuspid Spacer device in high-risk elderly patients, albeit limited in numbers, nevertheless points toward evidence of clinical safety and benefit, with patients showing objective improvements in functional capacity, sustained out to 1 year postprocedure. These findings are coupled with reduced evidence of the stigmata of right heart failure (less edema and lower diuretic dosages). Heart failure hospitalizations were also significantly reduced. These clinical findings were observed despite the absence of large, significant changes on echocardiographic

Table 4
One-year functional and laboratory outcomes

Outcome	Baseline (n = 18)	1 y (n = 14)[a]	P Value
NYHA grade	3.1 ± 0.5	2.0 ± 0.9	.0001
NYHA grade I/II	1 (6)	11 (79)	.0001
Hospitalization for heart failure[b]	10 (56)	1 (7)	.008
6-min walk test (m)	256 ± 103	328 ± 82	.04
Kansas City Cardiomyopathy Questionnaire score	63.0 ± 20.4	79.9 ± 22.4	.09
Edema score	1.9 ± 1.1	0.4 ± 0.7	.0001
Weight (kg)	74.1 ± 14.3	74.3 ± 16.5	.97
Daily furosemide dose (mg)	85 ± 73	73 ± 49	.6
B-type natriuretic peptide (pg/mL)	441 ± 432	NA	NA
N-terminal pro–B-type natriuretic peptide (pg/mL)	2812 ± 2798	2075 ± 1731	.39
eGFR (mL/min)	45.4 ± 16.7	49.5 ± 19.4	.52
Hemoglobin (g/dL)	11.8 ± 2.0	11.5 ± 1.9	.67

Values are mean ± SD or n (%). The P value was calculated for the comparison between baseline and 1-year results.
  [a] Data do not include 2 patients with failed procedures.
  [b] Baseline hospitalization events refers to the 12 months preceding the procedure.
  From Perlman G, Praz F, Puri R, et al. Transcatheter tricuspid valve repair with a new transcatheter coaptation system for the treatment of severe tricuspid regurgitation - one year clinical and echocardiographic results. JACC Cardiovasc Interv 2017; with permission.

imaging assessment of TR, in which many patients still showed moderate or moderate to severe TR despite functional improvement. Notably, most of these patients had torrential TR at baseline with severe tricuspid leaflet malcoaptation or noncoaptation.

These preliminary findings need to be considered within the context of the patient phenotype and disease substrate. Despite modest echocardiographic evidence of TR amelioration, clinicians need to consider the chronicity and severity of baseline TR and annular dilatation, and the inoperable state of the patients, to better place these findings into context. The enrolled patients represent the extreme end of the TR spectrum, whereby surgical intervention was prohibitive, and conventional medical therapies were unable to prevent repeated heart failure hospitalizations before FORMA insertion. As such, reducing baseline torrential TR to moderate to severe TR seemed to portend global, meaningful improvements in the functional and clinical status of the FORMA recipients. As such, insufficient coaptation after Spacer insertion proved difficult with the current limitations in sizes of available Spacers relative to the underlying pathologic substrate. Nevertheless, by comparison, the magnitude of benefit following FORMA implantation in the current cohort seemed to be similar to the preliminary benefits observed with various other experimental percutaneous therapies (ie, off-label MitraClip,

Trialign, Tricinch) to treat severe TR that partially corrected its severity.[7–9]

A further issue to arise from the early FORMA experience relates to the imaging assessment of TR severity, which remains a complex issue in the setting of a tricuspid Spacer device. Both quantitative and qualitative estimation of TR severity remain challenging given the effect that a Spacer device has on the underlying nature of the TR jets, which can be often further split into noncircular jets with a Spacer device placed in situ. Furthermore, the volume status and loading conditions of patients was likely variable, further influencing TR severity and variability. In addition, the propensity of the RV to remodel, as well as the possibility of variations in Spacer positioning over time, may ultimately contribute to ongoing variations in imaging assessment of TR with tricuspid Spacers. Further work needs to be conducted to ascertain the utility of complimentary imaging modalities in this setting (ie, cardiac MRI), the role of invasive hemodynamic monitoring, as well as that of serum biomarkers that could reflect atrial stretch before and after Spacer insertion. The device is MRI compatible.

Device thrombosis remains the Achilles heel of most, if not all, novel transcatheter-based prostheses for treating structural heart disorders. One patient showed FORMA device thrombosis in the setting of chronic subtherapeutic anticoagulation, remedied by

Table 5
One-year echocardiographic results

Variable	Baseline (n = 18)	1 y (n = 13)[a]	P Value
TR Grade			
None/trivial	0	0	1.0
Mild	0	1	.41
Moderate	0	2	.17
Moderate to severe	1	3	.28
Severe	6	4	1.0
Very severe[b]	11	3	.07
Severe/very severe	17	7	.01
EROA (mm^2)	103 ± 61	100 ± 52	.88
VC width (mm)	12.1 ± 3.9	8.3 ± 4.0	.01
Tricuspid annulus diameter (mm)	46.1 ± 6	42.1 ± 4.3	.049
RV Systolic Function[c]			
Normal	7	2	.22
Mildly reduced	7	3	.44
Moderately reduced	2	5	.18
Severely reduced	1	3	.29
RV Diameter, Base (mm)	55.1 ± 6.7	49.9 ± 4.7	.02
RV Diameter, midventricle (mm)	43.2 ± 7.4	41.6 ± 5.4	.52
RV systolic pressure (mm Hg)	43 ± 12	48 ± 19	.31
Inferior vena cava diameter (mm)	27 ± 7	24 ± 7	.26
RA volume (mL^2)	150 ± 58	133 ± 56	.43
Mitral regurgitation ≥ moderate	4 (22)	3 (28)	1.00
Left ventricle ejection fraction (%)	58 ± 9	58 ± 11	1.00

Values are mean ± SD or n (%). The P value was calculated for the comparison between baseline and 1-year results.
Abbreviation: RA, right atrium.
[a] Data do not include 2 patients with failed procedures; additionally, echocardiographic data were missing for 1 patient at 1 year.
[b] Very severe TR was categorized as a TR consistent with severe TR but with a VC greater than 12 mm or an EROA greater than 120 mm^2.
[c] Baseline imaging not sufficient for assessment of RV function in 1 patient.
From Perlman G, Praz F, Puri R, et al. Transcatheter tricuspid valve repair with a new transcatheter coaptation system for the treatment of severe tricuspid regurgitation - one year clinical and echocardiographic results. JACC Cardiovasc Interv 2017; with permission.

corrective dosing without major subsequent clinical sequelae. Nearly 90% of FORMA recipients presented with preexisting AF, necessitating underlying anticoagulation. However, in the absence of AF it remains unclear whether a period of systemic anticoagulation is required for patients undergoing Spacer implantation.

It is possible that device iterations could enable the broader applicability of Spacer devices for inoperable patients with moderate to severe tricuspid leaflet malcoaptation or noncoaptation. At present, the FORMA device is available in 12-mm and 15-mm sizes. The device is sized according to the following criteria: native tricuspid annulus area <2.14 cm^2 (9 mm device), <2.63 cm^2 (12 mm device) or <3.27 cm^2 (15 mm device) as measured by TTE or CT. The implementation of an 18-mm Spacer would potentially allow superior coaptation in patients presently treated with the 15-mm device who show multiple residual TR jets, as well as those with more dilated TV annuli. Furthermore, patients with pacemaker lead–induced TR represent a population with an unmet clinical need for effective therapies that could counteract the deleterious effects of a pacing lead contributing to TV leaflet malcoaptation. At present, patients with in situ pacemakers are potential FORMA candidates with the Spacer being positioned adjacent to the pacing lead across the TV, with venous access from the same side as the original pacemaker. Thus, most experience to date has been with patients possessing left-sided pacemakers. However, ongoing refinements in the FORMA delivery system could allow further experience to be gained in those with right-sided pacemakers, which currently present anatomic challenges for successful and safe FORMA device navigation. In addition, given the preponderance of pacemaker leads to provoke malcoaptation, and chronic RV pacing to further promote RV and ultimately TV annular dilatation,[10,11] pacemaker leads with inherent Spacerlike capabilities could facilitate a preemptive approach toward minimizing this iatrogenic, but underestimated, problem.

Two ongoing clinical registries in the United States and Europe will allow clinicians to better understand the efficacy of the FORMA device across a broader patient population. A US early feasibility study is currently ongoing (NCT02471807). It is planned to enroll 15 patients in the study with the primary outcome being procedural success, defined as successful device implantation with no device or procedural serious adverse events at 30 days. A larger trial was launched in the second half of 2016 (tricuSPid trAnsCatheter rEpaiR system [SPACER]; NCT02787408). The estimated enrollment consists of 75 patients, and the primary outcome assessed will be the cardiac mortality of the as-treated cohort at 30 days compared with a literature-derived performance goal based on high-risk surgical outcomes for tricuspid repair/replacement.

SUMMARY

At present, a percutaneous strategy for reducing TV leaflet noncoaptation or malcoaptation with a Spacer device (FORMA) seems safe, with evidence of early clinical efficacy sustained at 1 year in inoperable patients with severe TV annular dilatation and insufficiency. Although its efficacy in reducing TR was variable and modest, these changes seemed to translate into objective functional clinical benefits for most of the device recipients to date. However, ongoing registries will enroll larger patient numbers with longer follow-up periods to understand device performance better. Ultimately, randomized trials will be needed to provide definite data on the efficacy of the FORMA device for the treatment of this high-risk group of patients with severe symptomatic TR.

REFERENCES

1. Dreyfus GD, Martin RP, Chan KM, et al. Functional tricuspid regurgitation: a need to revise our understanding. J Am Coll Cardiol 2015; 65(21):2331–6.
2. Puri R, Rodes-Cabau J. Transcatheter interventions for tricuspid regurgitation: the FORMA repair system. EuroIntervention 2016;12(Y):Y113–5.
3. Campelo-Parada F, Perlman G, Philippon F, et al. First-in-man experience of a novel transcatheter repair system for treating severe tricuspid regurgitation. J Am Coll Cardiol 2015;66(22):2475–83.
4. Perlman G, Praz F, Puri R, et al. Transcatheter tricuspid valve repair with a new transcatheter coaptation system for the treatment of severe tricuspid regurgitation - one year clinical and echocardiographic results. JACC Cardiovasc Interv 2017. [Epub ahead of print].
5. Rudski LG, Lai WW, Afilalo J, et al. Guidelines for the echocardiographic assessment of the right heart in adults: a report from the American Society of Echocardiography endorsed by the European Association of Echocardiography, a registered branch of the European Society of Cardiology, and the Canadian Society of Echocardiography. J Am Soc Echocardiogr 2010;23(7):685–713 [quiz: 786–8].
6. Zoghbi WA, Adams D, Bonow RO, et al. Recommendations for noninvasive evaluation of native valvular regurgitation: a report from the American Society of Echocardiography developed in collaboration with the Society for Cardiovascular Magnetic Resonance. J Am Soc Echocardiogr 2017;30(4):303–71.
7. Latib A, Agricola E, Pozzoli A, et al. First-in-man implantation of a tricuspid annular remodeling device for functional tricuspid regurgitation. JACC Cardiovasc Interv 2015;8(13):e211–214.
8. Schofer J, Bijuklic K, Tiburtius C, et al. First-in-human transcatheter tricuspid valve repair in a patient with severely regurgitant tricuspid valve. J Am Coll Cardiol 2015;65(12):1190–5.
9. Hammerstingl C, Schueler R, Malasa M, et al. Transcatheter treatment of severe tricuspid regurgitation with the MitraClip system. Eur Heart J 2016;37(10):849–53.
10. Al-Bawardy R, Krishnaswamy A, Bhargava M, et al. Tricuspid regurgitation in patients with pacemakers and implantable cardiac defibrillators: a comprehensive review. Clin Cardiol 2013; 36(5):249–54.
11. Al-Mohaissen MA, Chan KL. Prevalence and mechanism of tricuspid regurgitation following implantation of endocardial leads for pacemaker or cardioverter-defibrillator. J Am Soc Echocardiogr 2012;25(3):245–52.

Caval Valve Implantation

Alexander Lauten, MD[a],[*], Henryk Dreger, MD[a], Michael Laule, MD[a],
Karl Stangl, MD[a], Hans R. Figulla, MD[b]

KEYWORDS

- Caval valve implantation • Tricuspid valve regurgitation • Tricuspid valve insufficiency
- Right heart failure • Functional tricuspid regurgitation

KEY POINTS

- Severe Tricuspid Regurgitation is associated with backflow into the caval veins which can result in significant morphologic alterations.
- Caval valve implantation (CAVI) results in resolution of venous backflow into the caval veins.
- Devices used for CAVI include the self-expandable TricValve and the ballon-expandable Edwards Sapien 3.

INTRODUCTION

Recently, transcatheter therapy has expanded the treatment options for patients with heart valve disease. Interventional therapy for aortic, mitral, and pulmonic valve disease is well established; however, catheter-based approaches to tricuspid regurgitation (TR) are still in early stages of development.[1–5] Traditionally, TR assumed a lower priority than other valve disease, also driven by less commercial interest in such developments in the past. Nevertheless, the prevalence and the functional impact of moderate to severe TR are high, and this disease is currently vastly undertreated.[6] With increasing severity of TR, 1-year mortality increases, reaching greater than 36% in those with severe TR.[7] Furthermore, the increasing number of patients at advanced age and high-risk profile undergoing successful treatment of left heart disease may contribute further to the growing need for effective interventional approaches of TR, because many of these potentially develop right heart disease at a later stage.[8,9]

For some of the interventional concepts to TR, including the edge-to-edge repair, transcatheter annuloplasty, the tricuspid spacer, and caval valves, procedural feasibility and favorable early clinical outcome have been demonstrated in small compassionate case series.[10–13] However, there is still a lack of evidence and data from randomized trials to demonstrate the functional impact of these treatment approaches. Furthermore, a better understanding of clinical and anatomic selection criteria for these approaches is needed as well as a uniform definition of achievable endpoints, which may differ depending on the subgroup of patients and treatment approaches.[14–16] This article reviews the pathophysiologic background and current evidence for caval valve implantation (CAVI) and examines the potential role of this approach for the treatment of severe TR.

Transcatheter Treatment of Tricuspid Regurgitation: Orthotopic versus Heterotopic Replacement

Although percutaneous repair concepts are conceptually attractive because they restore native tricuspid valve (TV) function, it remains arguable to which extent repair concepts can be implemented on the TV with durable long-term results. A repair procedure has to yield

---

Disclosure Statement: Consultant to P&F TricValve, receives research support from Edwards Lifesciences (A. Lauten). Consultant to P&F TricValve (H.R. Figulla).

[a] Department of Cardiology, Charité – Universitaetsmedizin Berlin, German Centre for Cardiovascular Research (DZHK), University Heart Center, Charitéplatz 1, Berlin D-10117, Germany; [b] University Heart Center Jena, Erlanger Allee 101, 07747 Jena, Germany
* Corresponding author.
E-mail address: alexander.lauten@charite.de

predictable and reproducible results in the hands of a wide range of interventional cardiologists to be adopted in clinical practice. Because of the above-mentioned unmet need for an effective treatment, transcatheter valve implantation may be an alternative and easier-to-achieve treatment option.

From the interventional perspective, there are 2 basic principles depending on the site of valve implantation: an *orthotopic* versus *heterotopic*, CAVI. For *orthotopic* valve replacement, the prosthetic valve is implanted in an anatomically correct position in the TV annulus, thus restoring the functional separation of the right ventricle (RV) and right atrium (RA). Although repair and heterotopic replacement tend to only partially correct TR, thus reducing the hemodynamic burden of acute complete correction to the RV, the orthotopic approach will most likely lead to complete correction of ventricular regurgitation. It remains arguable whether this is necessary to achieve clinical improvement or is hemodynamically desirable in patients with RV dysfunction.

Furthermore, the orthotopic approach is associated with particular challenges in patients with severe and long-standing TR. It was only recently that this approach was successfully performed for compassionate human treatment with an investigational device. Compared with the aortic annulus, the TV annulus offers a greater variability and less resistance for device fixation because of its larger diameter and lower proportion of fibrous tissue. Size and flexibility of the TV and the surrounding myocardium hamper positioning and long-term fixation of transcatheter devices, and there are no adjacent structures to facilitate implantation of such devices. Annulus dilatation may reach greater than 70 mm in functional TR and is associated with the loss of anatomic landmarks between RV and RA. A device intended for orthotopic TV replacement would require unique solutions for stent and catheter design as well as tissue valve engineering (eg, a 70-mm tissue valve would require a leaflet height of >40 mm to avoid prolapsing into the RA). In 2005, Boudjemline and colleagues[17] experimentally investigated this approach by means of implanting a double-disc nitinol stent with a semilunar valve into the TV annulus. Although in this study technical feasibility was demonstrated to some degree in healthy sheep, several difficulties relating to sufficient fixation of the self-expanding valve in the highly dynamic tricuspid annulus were observed.

Heterotopic CAVI is an obviously attractive alternative. Compared with the orthotopic approach, the heterotopic procedure benefits from the advantage of a straightforward implantation technique because of the distance to vulnerable cardiac structures. The introduction of foreign material in the RV inflow tract is avoided, permitting a potentially lower risk of injury to ventricular structures and making this an attractive approach to the interventional cardiologist. Devices do not interfere with any preexisting trans-tricuspid pacemaker or defibrillator leads, which might represent a limitation for orthotopic procedures on the TV.

The Caval Valve Implantation Approach: From Preclinical Proof-of-Concept to First Human Application

The CAVI concept was first investigated in an experimental study in animals demonstrating function and hemodynamic effects of the caval valves. After creation of acute TR in sheep, self-expanding valves were implanted in the inferior vena cava (IVC) and superior vena cava (SVC) using a transjugular approach (**Fig. 1**A). In this study, the onset of TR resulted in a significant reduction of cardiac output and a ventricular wave in the IVC. After implantation of the IVC and SVC valves, cardiac output and systolic backflow in the caval veins recovered to baseline value.[16,18] Chronic animal data demonstrated device function for a period of up to 6 months after implantation (see **Fig. 1**B, C).[19]

After demonstration of feasibility, CAVI was first applied for compassionate treatment in a human patient in 2010.[14] In this patient with severe functional TR after multiple preceding open-heart procedures, a self-expanding valve was implanted into the IVC at the cavoatrial junction to reduce regurgitant backflow. In this experience, excellent valve function was observed after deployment, resulting in a marked reduction of caval pressure and an abolition of backflow to the IVC (see **Fig. 1**D, E). The patient was discharged home and experienced an improvement of physical capacity and symptoms of right heart failure within the 3-month follow-up period.[20] The first series of patients treated with caval implantation of the Edwards Sapien XT valve (Edwards Lifesciences Inc, Irvine, CA, USA) was published by Laule and colleagues[21] in 2013, reporting the experience with IVC-implantation of balloon-expandable valves (BEV) in 3 patients with severe functional TR (see **Fig. 1**F, G).

Clinical Evidence

With the growing understanding of TR and its natural history, it becomes more and more obvious that this patient population is actually a heterogeneous cohort presenting for treatment in different stages of a continuous disease

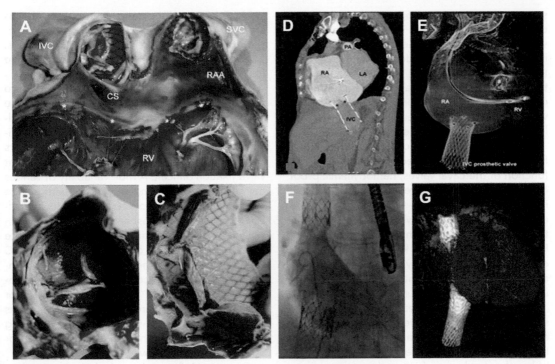

Fig. 1. From preclinical proof of concept to first human application. (*A–C*) Preclinical proof of concept was demonstrated in a sheep model of acute severe TR. The onset of TR resulted in a significant reduction of cardiac output and a ventricular wave in the IVC. After implantation of the IVC and SVC valves, cardiac output and systolic backflow in the caval veins recovered to baseline. Chronic animal data demonstrated device function for a period of up to 6 months after implantation. First-in-man demonstrated feasibility using custom-made devices for IVC only (*D, E*) and Edwards-Sapien XT valves for bicaval implantation (*F, G*). *, tricuspid valve; CS, coronary sinus; RAA, right atrial appendage.

process. It is yet unclear which interventional approach will result in a functional and clinical success and in which subtype of patient population. The various interventional approaches that are under development today, including edge-to-edge repair, annuloplasty, and the caval approach, potentially focus at different subgroups of TR patients and may also require different measures of outcome depending on disease stage.[12,13,22,23]

A recent observational study summarizes the current experience with CAVI in a multicenter series of 25 patients (Lauten A, Figulla HR, Sinning JM, et al. Transcatheter treatment of severe tricuspid regurgitationTR using caval valve implantation (CAVI), submitted for publication). The study demonstrates that treatment of severe TR with the CAVI technique is feasible, safe, and hemodynamically effective. Successful implantation of either self- expandable valves or BEV resulted in the resolution of caval backflow in all patients, and treatment further translated into New York Heart Association class improvement. However, with a mean Society of Thoracic Surgeons Score of 14.0 ± 12.7, the study included a high proportion of excessive risk patients and therefore observed a high 1-year mortality. This experience points out the importance of the selection of patients that may potentially benefit as well as the importance of definition of clinical or mortality endpoints.

Anatomic and Hemodynamic Patient Selection

Patients with significant TR may remain asymptomatic for many years. However, because TR frequently develops with the progression of left heart or pulmonary disease, the underlying disorder rather than the TV lesion tends to dominate the clinical picture. Increased right atrial pressure is transmitted to the central and hepatic veins, leading to hepatosplenomegaly and ascites, which are present in 90% of patients with severe TR.[6,24] In the advanced disease stage, TR and associated right heart failure are associated with a wide range of hemodynamic and anatomic alterations, including massive dilatation and elongation of the inferior and SVC. Because right ventricular stroke volume is partially expelled backwards into the venous system, there is a resulting decrease in cardiac output and RV afterload. This decrease in right ventricular afterload in the presence of TR may initially actually mask a decreased RV contractility. However, increasing volume overload contributes to further RV and tricuspid annulus dilatation, leading to a worsening of TR. As right ventricular preload increases, the RV further loses its contractility and eventually fails.

Pulsatile blood flow and systolic flow reversal in the caval veins are prerequisites for the proper function of the caval valves, hemodynamic proof of regurgitation is required before heterotopic implantation. Therefore, CAVI is likely to be effective only in patients with preserved RV function. The prognostic significance of preserved RV function is already known to affect the outcome after TV surgery and will probably to a certain degree also impact outcome after any interventional TV procedure.

When screening patients for CAVI, understanding the changes of venous anatomy associated with TR is of importance. In severe TR, the IVC dilates in the upper abdominal section below the diaphragm, frequently reaching diameters ~45 mm below the inflow of the hepatic veins. Because of the constraining outer fibrous structure of the crossing through the diaphragm, the uppermost IVC section hardly dilates. Thus, this section serves as preferred landing zone for secure valve implantation.

In contrast, the inflow section of the SVC into the RA tends to massively dilate, particularly the venous segment below the level of the right pulmonary artery. Dilatation of the SVC leads to atrialization of the distal venous segment and results in a tapered anatomy, which makes sufficient valve fixation difficult. A wide variability of venous diameters can be found in patients with severe TR, requiring dedicated devices that provide sufficient anchoring in most anatomies (**Fig. 2**).

Under the condition of severe TR, the anatomic diameter of the SVC and IVC frequently exceeds the suitable range for implantation of current commercially available devices. Regarding the Edwards Sapien XT or Sapien 3-Valve (Edwards Lifesciences), this has been partially compensated for by pre-stenting the caval veins before valve deployment for downsizing and improved valve anchoring.

Current CAVI experience includes the implantation of the balloon expandable Edwards

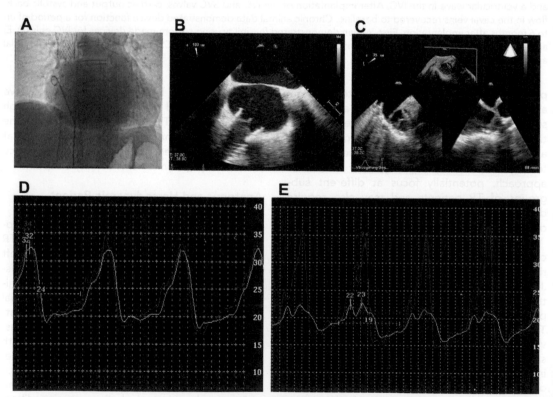

Fig. 2. Bicaval valve implantation using the self-expandable TricValve. (A–C) Fluoroscopy and transesophageal echocardiogram demonstrate the position and function of the dedicated devices in the SVC and IVC. Angiography (A) and invasive pressure tracings (D, E) confirm the complete resolution of caval backflow and a marked reduction of the V-wave and mean pressure in the IVC.

Sapien XT or Sapien 3 and the self-expandable TricValve (Product & Features, Vienna, Austria). Neither device is yet approved for venous implantation; all implantations have been performed under compassionate clinical use or within clinical study protocols.

Anatomic screening and decision for single versus bicaval implantation depended on the available devices. For implantation of BEV, an IVC diameter at the diaphragmatic intersection and an SVC diameter at the atrial inflow of ≤30 mm is suitable for valve implantation. Furthermore, a tapered anatomy or severe venous elongation of the SVC at the designated landing zone was considered unsuitable. Anatomic exclusion criteria for TricValve implantation include an IVC diameter at the diaphragmatic intersection and an SVC diameter at the SVC right pulmonary artery crossing of greater than 35 mm (Fig. 3).

How to Perform Caval Valve Implantation

Because of the commercial availability of the Edwards Sapien XT and Sapien 3 valves for treatment of aortic stenosis (29 mm Edwards Sapien XT or Sapien 3), there is a growing experience in the off-label use of these devices for CAVI. Although the use of BEV has been commonly limited to the IVC, in selected cases the long

segment of the SVC facilitates BEV implantation using the same implant technique. The anatomy of the cavoatrial junction of the IVC (particularly the large diameter, the inflow of hepatic veins, and the compliance of the venous wall) precludes direct implantation of a BEV and requires the preparation of a landing zone by implanting a self-expandable stent to facilitate valve fixation. Thus, a self-expandable stent tailored to IVC diameter (eg, 30 × 80 mm) is implanted in the IVC at the level of the diaphragm and protruding approximately 5 mm into the RA. The 29-mm BEV mounted on the delivery system is then deployed inside the stent with the lower part just superior to the confluence of the first hepatic vein.

The TricValve is designed as a set of 2 self-expandable valves dedicated for SVC and IVC implantation in the low-pressure circulation. The SVC valve is a belly-shaped tapered device for anchoring in dilated, tapered SVC configuration. The IVC valve is deployed at the level of the diaphragm and protruding into the RA. Both devices are made of bovine pericardium, and the inner part of the atrial stent portion is lined with a polytetrafluoroethylene skirt. Both valves are loaded into 27-French catheters for sheathless implantation. Before SVC valve implantation, a catheter is

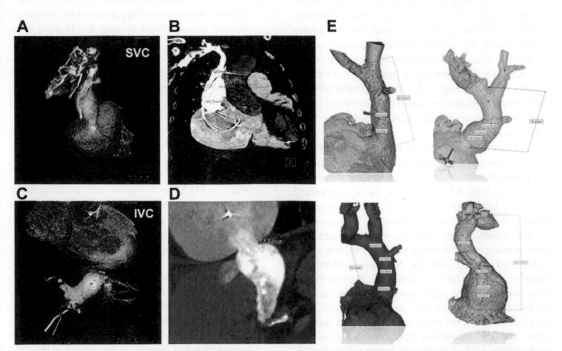

Fig. 3. Changes of venous anatomy associated with severe TR. Long-standing severe TR is associated with dilatation and elongation of the IVC and SVC with the diameter frequently exceeding the suitable range for implantation of current commercially available devices. The inflow section of the SVC into the RA massively dilates below the level of the right pulmonary artery (A, B, E). The IVC dilates in the upper abdominal section below the diaphragm but remains constrained by the diaphragm (C, D).

placed distally in the right pulmonary artery as marker of the IVC–right pulmonary artery (rPA) crossing. The SVC valve is then deployed with the landing zone of the enlarged midportion of the stent above the rPA. The IVC valve is deployed with the upper, skirt-lined segment of the stent protruding into the RA and the device fully deployed and anchored in the SVC.

Potential Limitations

Although CAVI is a rather simple procedure, this approach has important limitations currently restricting its use to nonsurgical patients with symptomatic TR in advanced-stage heart disease.

Nevertheless, limitations apply as well to heterotopic procedures. From a hemodynamic perspective, CAVI does not address TR itself, but the regurgitation of blood into the caval veins. As this condition is present only in a subgroup of patients with severe, often longstanding TR and RV enlargement, hemodynamic proof of caval regurgitation is essential before valve implantation. Also, it is yet unclear whether this subpopulation benefits from an interventional procedure. The persistence of right atrial volume overload and the ventricularization of the RA are potential limitations of the procedure, and its long-term impact on right atrial and ventricular function is currently unknown. Although follow-up data in small patient series demonstrate no further RA enlargement up to 12 month after implantation, further evaluation with long-term follow-up is required (Lauten A, Figulla HR, Sinning JM, et al. Transcatheter treatment of severe tricuspid regurgitation using caval valve implantation (CAVI), submitted for publication).

Furthermore, CAVI addresses the regurgitation of blood in the caval veins only, a condition not found in every patient with severe TR. In this condition, the RA functions as a compliant reservoir by retaining part of the regurgitant volume and thus limiting systolic flow reversal in the caval veins. Therefore, only patients with proven systolic flow reversal in the caval veins and preserved RV function potentially benefit from this treatment. Furthermore, symptoms of right heart congestion are caused by elevation of mean IVC pressure, which may be slightly reduced after CAVI. Current experience shows, however, that because of RV dysfunction and elevation of mean RA pressure, vena cava pressure is not normalized after CAVI but still remains elevated, which also limits the hemodynamic and functional benefit of the procedure.

SUMMARY

For a large number of patients with functional TR in an advanced stage of multivalvular heart disease, a readily available transcatheter approach could offer an effective treatment option. Their number is likely to increase in the future because of the demographic development and the widespread application of interventional therapies for left heart valve disease. In carefully selected patients, CAVI is a technically straightforward interventional technique and has been applied successfully for compassionate treatment in human patients. Hemodynamic improvement has been consistently observed; however, the clinical benefit of the procedure still requires further evaluation, and important hemodynamic limitations apply. As for any other treatment concept of TR, it remains to be determined which patients benefit most from this approach and which outcome measures are most suitable.

REFERENCES

1. Leon MB, Smith CR, Mack MJ, et al. Transcatheter or surgical aortic-valve replacement in intermediate-risk patients. N Engl J Med 2016;374:1609–20.
2. Figulla HR, Webb JG, Lauten A, et al. The transcatheter valve technology pipeline for treatment of adult valvular heart disease. Eur Heart J 2016; 37:2226–39.
3. Lauten A, Figulla HR, Mollmann H, et al. TAVI for low-flow, low-gradient severe aortic stenosis with preserved or reduced ejection fraction: a subgroup analysis from the German Aortic Valve Registry (GARY). EuroIntervention 2014;10:850–9.
4. Latib A, Mangieri A, Agricola E, et al. Percutaneous bicuspidalization of the tricuspid valve using the MitraClip system. Int J Cardiovasc Imaging 2017; 33:227–8.
5. Möllmann H, Linke A, Holzhey DM, et al. Implantation and 30-day follow-up on all 4 valve sizes within the portico transcatheter aortic bioprosthetic family. JACC Cardiovasc Interv 2017;10(15):1538–47.
6. Stuge O, Liddicoat J. Emerging opportunities for cardiac surgeons within structural heart disease. J Thorac Cardiovasc Surg 2006;132:1258–61.
7. Nath J, Foster E, Heidenreich PA. Impact of tricuspid regurgitation on long-term survival. J Am Coll Cardiol 2004;43:405–9.
8. Rogers JH, Bolling SF. The tricuspid valve: current perspective and evolving management of tricuspid regurgitation. Circulation 2009;119:2718–25.
9. Selle A, Figulla HR, Ferrari M, et al. Impact of rapid ventricular pacing during TAVI on microvascular tissue perfusion. Clin Res Cardiol 2014;103:902–11.

10. Rodes-Cabau J, Hahn RT, Latib A, et al. Transcatheter therapies for treating tricuspid regurgitation. J Am Coll Cardiol 2016;67:1829–45.

11. Campelo-Parada F, Perlman G, Philippon F, et al. First-in-man experience of a novel transcatheter repair system for treating severe tricuspid regurgitation. J Am Coll Cardiol 2015;66:2475–83.

12. Schofer J, Bijuklic K, Tiburtius C, et al. First-in-human transcatheter tricuspid valve repair in a patient with severely regurgitant tricuspid valve. J Am Coll Cardiol 2015;65:1190–5.

13. Nickenig G, Kowalski M, Hausleiter J, et al. Transcatheter treatment of severe tricuspid regurgitation with the edge-to-edge mitraclip technique. Circulation 2017;135:1802–14.

14. Lauten A, Ferrari M, Hekmat K, et al. Heterotopic transcatheter tricuspid valve implantation: first-in-man application of a novel approach to tricuspid regurgitation. Eur Heart J 2011;32:1207–13.

15. Mangieri A, Montalto C, Pagnesi M, et al. Mechanism and implications of the tricuspid regurgitation: from the pathophysiology to the current and future therapeutic options. Circ Cardiovasc Interv 2017;10 [pii:e005043].

16. Lauten A, Figulla HR, Willich C, et al. Percutaneous caval stent valve implantation: investigation of an interventional approach for treatment of tricuspid regurgitation. Eur Heart J 2010;31:1274–81.

17. Boudjemline Y, Agnoletti G, Bonnet D, et al. Steps toward the percutaneous replacement of atrioventricular valves an experimental study. J Am Coll Cardiol 2005;46:360–5.

18. Lauten A, Figulla HR, Willich C, et al. Heterotopic valve replacement as an interventional approach to tricuspid regurgitation. J Am Coll Cardiol 2010;55:499–500.

19. Lauten A, Laube A, Schubert H, et al. Transcatheter treatment of tricuspid regurgitation by caval valve implantation–experimental evaluation of decellularized tissue valves in central venous position. Catheter Cardiovasc Interv 2015;85:150–60.

20. Lauten A, Hamadanchi A, Doenst T, et al. Caval valve implantation for treatment of tricuspid regurgitation: post-mortem evaluation after mid-term follow-up. Eur Heart J 2014;35:1651.

21. Laule M, Stangl V, Sanad W, et al. Percutaneous transfemoral management of severe secondary tricuspid regurgitation with Edwards Sapien XT bioprosthesis: first-in-man experience. J Am Coll Cardiol 2013;61:1929–31.

22. Rosser BA, Taramasso M, Maisano F. Transcatheter interventions for tricuspid regurgitation: TriCinch (4Tech). EuroIntervention 2016;12:Y110–2.

23. Latib A, Agricola E, Pozzoli A, et al. First-in-man implantation of a tricuspid annular remodeling device for functional tricuspid regurgitation. JACC Cardiovasc Interv 2015;8:e211–4.

24. Singh JP, Evans JC, Levy D, et al. Prevalence and clinical determinants of mitral, tricuspid, and aortic regurgitation (the Framingham Heart Study). Am J Cardiol 1999;83:897–902.

Transcatheter Tricuspid Valve Replacement

Amar Krishnaswamy, MD[a],*, Jose Navia, MD[b], Samir R. Kapadia, MD[c]

KEYWORDS

- Tricuspid regurgitation • Tricuspid valve • Transcatheter tricuspid valve replacement
- Tricuspid bioprosthesis degeneration

KEY POINTS

- Tricuspid valve-in-valve procedures demonstrate good results and can be performed in a relatively straightforward manner.
- Tricuspid valve-in-ring procedures demonstrate reasonable efficacy, but operators should be facile in treating paravalvular leak which is common after the ViR procedure.
- Newer technologies and device development for replacement of native tricuspid valve pathology are under development and investigation, though none are currently available for commercial use.

INTRODUCTION

Tricuspid regurgitation (TR) is a common entity, most commonly functional in nature due to right-sided dysfunction in the setting of concomitant cardiac disease or pulmonary hypertension. Patients living with TR often experience numerous limitations as a result of right-sided heart failure symptoms, including functional decline, frequent hospitalizations, liver failure, and kidney failure. Furthermore, patients with significant TR demonstrate worse survival, although a cause-and-effect relationship has not been proven.

Transcatheter techniques to either repair or replace the tricuspid valve (TV) are a burgeoning frontier in structural cardiac interventions. Numerous devices are currently in preclinical and early-feasibility stages. In this review, the authors discuss the current landscape of transcatheter TV replacement (TTVR), with other articles devoted to percutaneous TV repair (TVRe) techniques.

PATIENT SELECTION

Appropriate patient selection is a key element for all invasive procedures. In contemporary surgical practice, patients undergoing surgery for coronary artery bypass or other valve disease often undergo concomitant TVRe in the setting either of severe TR, or if the annulus is dilated >40 mm, as a preemptive strategy. This scenario represents the majority (87%) of TV surgical procedures. Conversely, isolated TVRe is rarer, constituting 13% of TV surgeries.[1]

This surgical practice of "incidental" TVre/replacement does not provide much guidance to the new field of TTVR. Because the clinical consequences of TR with regard to survival are unclear, preemptive TTVR for native TR is likely a bridge-too-far in the current early era of these devices that are simply trying to establish technical feasibility. On the other hand, for patients whose symptoms of severe TR are not

[a] Section of Interventional Cardiology, Department of Cardiovascular Medicine, Heart and Vascular Institute, Cleveland Clinic, 9500 Euclid Avenue, Cleveland, OH 44195, USA; [b] Department of Cardiothoracic Surgery, Heart and Vascular Institute, Cleveland Clinic, 9500 Euclid Avenue, Cleveland, OH 44195, USA; [c] Interventional Cardiology, Sones Cardiac Catheterization Laboratory, Heart and Vascular Institute, Cleveland Clinic, 9500 Euclid Avenue, Cleveland, OH 44195, USA
* Corresponding author.
E-mail address: akrishnaswamy@gmail.com

Intervent Cardiol Clin 7 (2018) 65–70
https://doi.org/10.1016/j.iccl.2017.08.009
2211-7458/18/© 2017 Elsevier Inc. All rights reserved.

controlled with medical heart failure therapies, and who are willing to consider early-phase clinical use, TTVR may be a reasonable choice when a thorough conversation regarding risks and benefits has been had. However, even for these patients, it is important to fully understand pulmonary hemodynamics and right ventricular mechanics, because patients with long-standing and severe pulmonary hypertension or right ventricular dysfunction may not benefit from TTVR despite a technically successful valve replacement.

It is most important that clinical trials of new devices for TTVR account for these limitations in their inclusion/exclusion criteria and endpoints. Even among the limited data available thus far in trials of percutaneous TVre or implantation of transcatheter aortic valve prosthetics in either TV rings or valves, there is little information provided about specific anatomic selection or right-sided mechanics.[2–4] Moving forward for studies of new treatments for TR, it is necessary that trials carefully standardize and report patient selection criteria, echocardiographic screening of right-sided parameters, device-specific anatomic selection factors, and objective clinical and echocardiographic outcomes so that the best use can be made of the trial data to inform future practice and applications.[5]

Patients with a degenerated surgical ring repair or bioprosthetic TV replacement are also an important group. In both of these situations, investigators have demonstrated (in mostly small case series) the use of currently available transcatheter aortic valve replacement (TAVR) devices for the valve-in-valve (ViV) or valve-in-ring (ViR) application. As discussed earlier, the degree of pulmonary disease and right-sided dysfunction must be carefully assessed and physicians must come to an understanding regarding the contribution of the TR to the patient's functional decline and the likelihood of clinical success with placement of a TAVR prosthesis in the degenerated surgical repair/replacement. If the TV surgery was performed in conjunction with other valve surgery, it is also important to make sure that the TV is the only prosthesis that is severely degenerated or contributing to symptoms. In appropriately selected patients, these ViV and ViR procedures are performed in an off-label fashion.

VALVE-IN-RING REPLACEMENT FOR PRIOR TRICUSPID VALVE REPAIR

As noted in earlier discussion, several patients undergo TV ring repair in the setting of symptomatic severe TR or incidentally as part of another cardiac surgery in selected situations. In recent years, approximately 9000 patients undergo TV surgery annually.[6] As noted previously, almost 90% of those surgeries are repairs. The surgical literature has been reasonably consistent in demonstrating the superiority of ring annuloplasty over suture-based techniques alone with regard to TR recurrence.[7] Nevertheless, over time, these repairs may degenerate and leave the patient with severe TR that is symptomatically poorly tolerated. By 8 years postoperatively, more than one-third of patients have 3 to 4+ TR.[8] A repeat cardiac surgery for isolated severe TR is rarely undertaken given the generally high-risk nature of the surgery of the patients and resultant poor outcomes.[9]

Placement of catheter-valve prostheses in a ViR fashion is therefore often considered for these patients and can provide important functional benefit (**Fig. 1**). The largest series of tricuspid valve-in-ring (TViR) implantation was recently published by Aboulhosn and colleagues.[3] Of 22 patients planned for TViR, 20 (91%) ultimately underwent valve implantation. Of these 20 patients, 17 had a SAPIEN valve (Edwards Lifesciences, Irvine, CA, USA) implanted and 3 had a Melody valve (Medtronic Inc, Minneapolis, MN, USA). Most (16/20, 73%) were implanted via the femoral venous route. Despite the high-risk nature of the group (patients on average had undergone 2 prior cardiac surgeries), the overall results were reasonable with no procedural mortality.

With regard to efficacy, no patients were left with valvular tricuspid stenosis (TS) or TR, although 15 patients (75%) had some degree of paravalvular leak (PVL). Nine of these were trivial or mild, 4 were moderate, and 2 were severe. Significant PVL was most often (78%) located in the "open" medial aspect of the incomplete ring. Including during the index TViR procedure, 6 patients had device closure of the PVL; 1 patient had multiple TViR placed but ultimately underwent surgery, and 1 patient went to surgery 6 days after the index TViR for severe PVL. Whereas almost 90% of patients had New York Heart Association (NYHA) III or IV symptoms at preprocedure, the investigators report that "most patients" had improvement in functional capacity after TViR.

Another important insight from this small series is the understanding that not all rings respond similarly to TViR procedures. For instance, most rings in current use are incomplete rigid or semi-rigid ovals, which may not be well deformed by a round catheter valve.

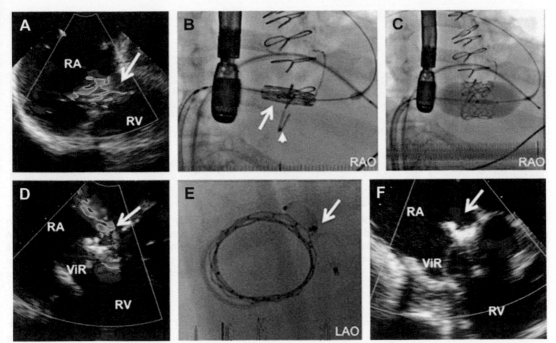

Fig. 1. Transcatheter tricuspid ViR implantation and PVL closure. (*A*) Severe valvular TR (*arrow*); (*B*) balloon-expandable TAVR in position (*arrow*) within the tricuspid ring (*arrowhead*); (*C*) valve deployment; (*D*) severe PVL in the area of the incomplete tricuspid ring (*arrow*); (*E*) 2 Amplatzer vascular plug II devices in the paravalvular space (*arrow*); (*F*) trivial residual PVL (*arrow*). LAO, left anterior oblique; RA, right atrium; RAO, right anterior oblique; RV, right ventricle.

The incomplete portion of the ring is placed at the apex of the triangle of Koch to minimize atrioventicular node trauma and conduction damage. Unfortunately, placement of a valve in the incomplete ring in the present series often resulted in PVL at this medial "open" aspect of the ring, as seen in the patient in **Fig. 1**. This is also the region where further leaflet tethering (septal leaflet) occurs over time in patients with functional TR and could result in worsening of PVL in the future even if only minimal or treated at the index procedure. Thankfully, as interventionalists and surgeons continue to work closely together in the structural heart disease space, newer ring designs are under development that could facilitate both surgical approaches and future ViR treatments in the future.[10]

VALVE-IN-VALVE REPLACEMENT FOR BIOPROSTHETIC TRICUSPID VALVE DEGENERATION

Just less than 1000 patients in the United States undergo TVR using a bioprosthesis placement annually.[6] Although TVre using ring annuloplasty is the favored approach, those patients whose valve is too remodeled for repair have significant leaflet tethering or severe right ventricular dilation, or who have failed prior TVre may require TVR.[11] An accurate estimate of TVR longevity is difficult to know, because "freedom from reoperation" statistics likely underestimate the true incidence of valve degeneration because reoperation for isolated TV disease is rare and carries a high degree of surgical risk. Nevertheless, in clinical practice it is not uncommon to see patients who are functionally limited due to severe bioprosthetic TR or TS. For appropriately selected patients, tricuspid valve-in-valve (TViV) implantation can often be performed effectively and with limited procedural risk (**Fig. 2**).

Reporting of TViV procedures, similar to TViR procedures, is generally limited to small case series of a few patients.[12] The largest series of TViV implantation was reported in the Valve-in-Valve International Database registry and enrolled patients between 2008 and 2015.[4] Of the 152 patients in whom TViV was attempted, 94 had a Melody valve (Medtronic Inc) and 58 had an Edwards SAPIEN series valve. The Melody patients were generally younger (average age 27 vs 53 years), were more likely than the SAPIEN patients to have congenital (67% vs 36%) than acquired TV disease (33% vs 64%), and on

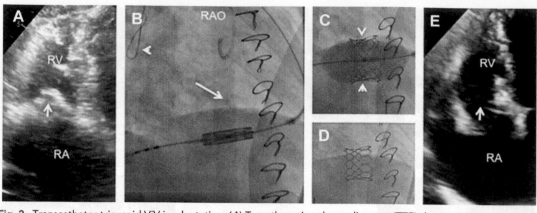

Fig. 2. Transcatheter tricuspid ViV implantation. (*A*) Transthoracic echocardiogram (TTE) demonstrates severe bioprosthetic TVR leaflet calcification and tricuspid stenosis (*arrow*); (*B*) balloon-expandable TAVR in position within the TVR annulus (*arrow*) and the Amplatz extra-stiff wire in the distal right pulmonary artery (*arrowhead*); (*C*) valve deployment; note the waist as the valve is oversized to provide stability within the annulus (*arrowheads*); (*D*) ViV in place; (*E*) TTE demonstrates large TV ViV orifice (*arrow*). LAO, left anterior oblique; RA, right atrium; RAO, right anterior oblique.

average had a smaller diameter TV bioprosthetic. Perhaps reflecting the earlier era of transcatheter valve procedures, 90% of cases were performed under general anesthesia. Most patients (69%) had transfemoral access; a minority was performed via the jugular route (28%), and a handful was performed via surgical right atrial access (3%). Of the entire group, 1 failed implantation because of inability to cross the TVR and 2 had valve embolization that were retrieved to the inferior vena cava; one of these patients had a successful TViV during the procedure and the other underwent surgical TVR 5 months later. A total of 4 patients had poor TViV hemodynamics (2 with moderate TR and 2 with moderate TS), 1 had moderate PVL, and 7 had mild PVL. Important 30-day outcomes include 5 deaths (0.03%), 1 of which was procedurally related, and improvement of at least 1 NYHA class among 76% (with 87% in NYHA I or II).

Ruparelia and colleagues,[13] using the newest generation Edwards SAPIEN-3 valve that is designed with a more flexible catheter and a sealing skirt to minimize PVL, reported the most contemporary series of TViV placement. They successfully performed TViV in 5 patients via the transfemoral route under conscious sedation. All patients had a 29-mm valve implanted; no patients had PVL; 1 patient had mild valvular TR, and there were no deaths within 30 days.

NATIVE TRICUSPID VALVE DISEASE

As discussed earlier, native TV regurgitation is usually treated in patients undergoing cardiac

surgery for other reasons, whether the regurgitation is severe or if it is moderate with evidence of TV annulus dilation. On the other hand, isolated TV surgery is relatively rare, especially for those patients who develop severe and symptomatic TR at some point after prior cardiac surgery. Among patients who do undergo isolated TV surgery, whether as a first-time operation or as a re-do, operative mortality approaches 10%.[14] An alternative to traditional cardiac surgery would therefore be readily welcomed by patients and surgeons alike.

Catheter valve implantation in the tricuspid position has several challenges. Anatomically, the TV annulus is not as fibrous and rigid as the mitral position (and certainly much less so than the aortic position). The TV annulus is also quite large, thereby requiring a larger device. In patients with longstanding TV disease and right-sided chamber dilation, this provides an even greater obstacle to percutaneous device placement. Replacement of the native TV in patients using transcatheter methods has been performed in limited numbers using existing valve platforms. As the interventional community's interest in the TV has been slowly increasing, however, newer designs are in various stages of development.

The first report of a catheter valve implanted in a native TV was published by Kefer and colleagues.[15] A 47-year-old woman with congenital cardiac disease and multiple prior cardiac surgeries including 3 prior suture-based tricuspid repairs without ring annuloplasty presented with severe TR and TS. Under support with extracorporeal membrane oxygenation,

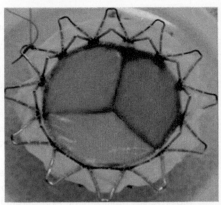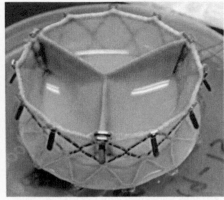

Fig. 3. Navigate self-expanding TV prosthesis. (*Courtesy of* NaviGate Cardiac Structures, Inc, Lake Forest, CA; with permission.)

the TV annulus was prestented using two 34-mm CP-covered stents (NuMED, Hopkinton, NY, USA) mounted on a 30-mm Crystal balloon (Balt, Montmorency, France). A 26-mm Edwards SAPIEN XT valve was then deployed within the stented segment. Because of significant PVL as a result of a too-ventricular position of the valve, a second SAPIEN XT was deployed more atrially with abolition of the PVL and good hemodynamics. The procedure was complicated by branch pulmonary artery perforation by the stiff wire, which was treated using coil embolization. The patient was hemodynamically and clinically well at 5-month follow-up.

The authors' group has recently been involved in native TV catheter-based valve replacement using the novel Navigate valve system, developed by Cleveland Clinic cardiac surgeon, Jose Navia. Two patients have been successfully treated thus far under US Food and Drug Administration compassionate use device exemption. The first was treated via right thoracotomy because of a chronically occluded internal jugular (IJ) vein; the second patient was treated via the right IJ (**Fig. 3**). As of this writing, an article describing these 2 cases in greater detail is in preparation. Other valve designs are in development along with trials of balloon-expandable TAVR deployment in the vena cava and placement of the Tric Valve device (P&F Products & Features Vertriebs GmbH, in cooperation with Braìle Biomedica) which consists of 2 self-expanding bioprostheses in the vena cava.

SUMMARY

Patients with significant tricuspid disease, whether native valve, with prior TV ring annuloplasty, or within a prior TV replacement often present with significant symptoms but may not be ideal candidates for operation or reoperation. As always, it will be important to develop a better understanding of which patients can be helped and which patients may be beyond help as a result of poor right-sided mechanics or comorbid conditions. Although there are limitations to the currently available transcatheter options for the patients, the initial data demonstrate the relative safety of using existing devices with good results and functional improvement. The best studied is TViV for patients with prior TVR, and more recent experience with the newest generation SAPIEN-3 valve is quite promising. Devices for native TR currently in development may herald a new era for the treatment of patients without prior TV surgery.

REFERENCES

1. Kilic A, Saha-Chaudhuri P, Rankin JS, et al. Trends and outcomes of tricuspid valve surgery in North America: an analysis of more than 50,000 patients from the Society of Thoracic Surgeons database. Ann Thorac Surg 2013;96:1546–52 [discussion: 1552].
2. Nickenig G, Kowalski M, Hausleiter J, et al. Transcatheter treatment of severe tricuspid regurgitation with the edge-to-edge mitraclip technique. Circulation 2017;135:1802–14.
3. Aboulhosn J, Cabalka AK, Levi DS, et al. Transcatheter valve-in-ring implantation for the treatment of residual or recurrent tricuspid valve dysfunction after prior surgical repair. JACC Cardiovasc Interv 2017;10:53–63.
4. McElhinney DB, Cabalka AK, Aboulhosn JA, et al, Valve-in-Valve International Database Registry. Transcatheter tricuspid valve-in-valve implantation for the treatment of dysfunctional surgical bioprosthetic valves: an international, multicenter registry study. Circulation 2016;133:1582–93.

5. Kapadia S, Krishnaswamy A, Tuzcu EM. Percutaneous therapy for tricuspid regurgitation: a new frontier for interventional cardiology. Circulation 2017;135:1815–8.

6. STS Adult Cardiac Surgery Database 2016. Available at: http://wwwstsorg/sites/default/files/documents/2016Harvest2_ExecutiveSummary_newpdf. Accessed August 6, 2017.

7. Parolari A, Barili F, Pilozzi A, et al. Ring or suture annuloplasty for tricuspid regurgitation? A meta-analysis review. Ann Thorac Surg 2014;98:2255–63.

8. McCarthy PM, Bhudia SK, Rajeswaran J, et al. Tricuspid valve repair: durability and risk factors for failure. J Thorac Cardiovasc Surg 2004;127:674–85.

9. Jeganathan R, Armstrong S, Al-Alao B, et al. The risk and outcomes of reoperative tricuspid valve surgery. Ann Thorac Surg 2013;95:119–24.

10. McCarthy PM. Valve-in-ring and the forgotten valve. JACC Cardiovasc Interv 2017;10:64–5.

11. Starck CT, Kempfert J, Falk V. Tricuspid valve interventions: surgical techniques and outcomes. EuroIntervention 2015;11(Suppl W):W128–32.

12. Raval J, Nagaraja V, Eslick GD, et al. Transcatheter valve-in-valve implantation: a systematic review of literature. Heart Lung Circ 2014;23:1020–8.

13. Ruparelia N, Mangieri A, Ancona M, et al. Percutaneous transcatheter treatment for tricuspid bioprosthesis failure. Catheter Cardiovasc Interv 2016;88:994–1001.

14. Ejiofor JI, Neely RC, Yammine M, et al. Surgical outcomes of isolated tricuspid valve procedures: repair versus replacement. Ann Cardiothorac Surg 2017;6:214–22.

15. Kefer J, Sluysmans T, Vanoverschelde JL. Transcatheter Sapien valve implantation in a native tricuspid valve after failed surgical repair. Catheter Cardiovasc Interv 2014;83:841–5.

Section 2: Interventional Therapy for Pulmonary Embolism

PREFACE

The Evolving State of Care for Acute Pulmonary Embolism

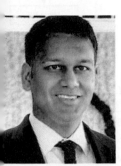

Jay Giri, MD, MPH
Editor

Pulmonary embolism (PE) is the world's third leading cardiovascular cause of death. Despite this, and in stark contrast to myocardial infarction and acute stroke, relatively little research has been devoted to novel pharmacologic or endovascular approaches to diminish the mortality and morbidity associated with acute PE. Comprehensive centers specializing in myocardial infarction care and stroke care have proliferated with the goal of providing urgent revascularization to patients suffering from these conditions. There have been comparatively few efforts to establish such novel health care delivery efforts in the care of acute PE. Recently, this has changed with the emergence of the "pulmonary embolism response team" model of care that aims to provide urgent multidisciplinary care to patients suffering from intermediate- or high-risk PE.

Part of the reason for the historic discrepancy in how PE is handled owes to a difference in pathophysiology of the disease process. In myocardial infarction and stroke, time is myocardium or brain. Infarction of these tissues leads to largely irreversible damage that has impact on both short- and long-term clinical outcomes. With PE, time is not lung. The most important pathophysiologic effect of PE that drives symptoms owes to an indirect effect on the right ventricle, which faces an acutely raised afterload. Observational data reveal that the majority of patients who present with PE will improve dramatically with isolated anticoagulation without experiencing long-term cardiopulmonary consequences of their acute event. However, important minorities of patients suffer acute mortality or long-term consequences of the disease with development of dyspneic syndromes or clinically significant chronic thromboembolic pulmonary hypertension.

The variability in prognosis for the acute PE event leads to difficult decision making. This complexity is often heightened in the face of a variety of patient comorbidities. Patients who may experience sequelae of PE represent an appealing target for interventional therapies to reduce this incidence. Currently, little comparative data exist to guide decision making around the use of endovascular therapies in PE. There is no question this should be a priority of medical research going forward. In the absence of data, individual centers must develop their own treatment guidelines for utilization of a variety of therapies for PE (**Fig. 1**).

The current issue seeks to clarify the state of endovascular therapies for PE, summarizing both the risks and benefits of therapies (often based on fairly low-quality evidence) and providing concrete technical advice on how to perform procedures when they are judged to have potential for

Intervent Cardiol Clin 7 (2018) xv–xvi
https://doi.org/10.1016/j.iccl.2017.10.002
2211-7458/18/© 2017 Published by Elsevier Inc.

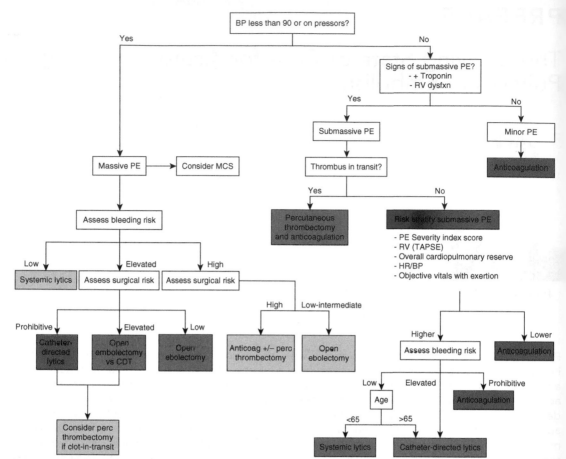

Fig. 1. Algorithm for intermediate and high risk PE at the University of Pennsylvania. BP, blood pressure; CDT, catheter-directed thrombolysis; dysfxn, dysfunction; HR, heart rate; MCS, mechanical circulatory support; perc., percutaneous; RV, right ventricle; TAPSE, tricuspid annular plane systolic excursion.

improving outcomes. The issue largely applies only to the patient with intermediate- or high-risk PE, as low-risk PE is best treated with isolated anticoagulation.

In our first article, Dr Chatterjee and colleagues review the fairly extensive literature related to utilization of systemic thrombolysis for PE. This leads to subsequent articles discussing interventional alternatives to this therapy, including catheter-directed thrombolysis by Dr Sista and colleagues and catheter-directed embolectomy by Dr Jaber and colleagues. Dr Mahmud and colleagues offer a fascinating discussion on balloon pulmonary angioplasty for chronic thromboembolic pulmonary hypertension, a technique that is in its embryonic stages in the United States. A technical review by Dr Elder and colleagues of acute mechanical circulatory support with classic extracorporeal membrane oxygen and novel percutaneous right ventricular support devices follows. And finally, Dr Kaufman and colleagues discuss the current state of inferior vena cava filters for PE.

Jay Giri, MD, MPH
Perelman School of Medicine
Interventional Cardiology &
Vascular Medicine
Division of Cardiovascular Medicine
University of Pennsylvania
3400 Civic Center Boulevard
Perelman Center South Tower, 11-105
Philadelphia, PA 19102, USA

E-mail address:
giri.jay@gmail.com

Systemic Thrombolysis for Pulmonary Embolism
Evidence, Patient Selection, and Protocols for Management

Hafeez Ul Hassan Virk, MD[a,1], Sanjay Chatterjee, MD[b,2],
Partha Sardar, MD[c,3], Chirag Bavishi, MD, MPH[a,4],
Jay Giri, MD, MPH[d], Saurav Chatterjee, MD[e,*,5]

KEYWORDS

- Pulmonary embolism • Systemic thrombolysis • Selection of patients • Risk stratification
- Management protocol

KEY POINTS

- Acute pulmonary embolism is associated with significant morbidity and mortality.
- Treatment options include anticoagulation, systemic thrombolysis, catheter-based interventions, and surgical embolectomy.
- Selecting candidates who derive maximal benefit with thrombolysis, while being exposed to the least possible risks of bleeding is difficult.
- Optimal and pragmatic selection of patients should involve a multidisciplinary approach.

INTRODUCTION

Pulmonary embolism (PE) affects 23 per 100,000 people annually,[1] causing morbidity including prolonged hospital stay, recurrence, postthrombotic syndrome, and even mortality. Annual US mortality rates associated with PE are 4 to 5 times greater than those associated with breast cancer or human immunodeficiency virus.[1,2] The incidence of PE rises with increasing age with an associated 1-year mortality approaching 39% in the elderly.[3] It affects hospitalized patients as well as outpatients, with an in-hospital fatality rate of 12%.[1] In spite of recent advances in diagnostic tools, PE remains underdiagnosed and is still considered a diagnostic dilemma, presenting with a wide range of symptoms from mild dyspnea to sudden death. Depending on the likelihood of PE, initial diagnostic tests include D-Dimer, electrocardiogram, cardiac biomarkers, transthoracic echocardiography, computed tomography (CT) scans, and

Disclosure: None (for all authors).
[a] Mount Sinai St Luke's-Roosevelt Hospitals, 1111 Amsterdam Avenue, 3rd Floor, Clark Building, New York, NY 10025, USA; [b] Apollo Gleneagles Hospital, 58, Canal Circular Road, Kolkata, West Bengal 700054, India; [c] Division of Cardiovascular Medicine, University of Utah, 30 North 1900 East, Room 4A100, Salt Lake City, UT 84132, USA; [d] Penn Cardiovascular Outcomes, Quality and Evaluative Research Center, 3400 Civic Center Boulevard, Philadelphia, PA 19104, USA; [e] Hoffman Heart Institute, Saint Francis Hospital, University of Connecticut School of Medicine, 110 Woodland Street, Hartford, CT 06106, USA
[1] Present address: #9 to 210 Apartment, Chestnut Hill Village Apartments, 7800 Stenton Avenue, Philadelphia, PA 19118.
[2] Present address: 1010 Arch Street Apartment 604, Philadelphia, PA 19107.
[3] Present address: 66 South Main Street Apartment 480, Salt Lake City, UT 84101.
[4] Present address: 515 West, 59th Street Apartment 27F, New York, NY 10019.
[5] Present address: 1010 Arch Street Apartment 604, Philadelphia, PA 19107.
* Corresponding author.
E-mail address: sauravchatterjeemd@gmail.com

ventilation perfusion scans. Based on the results of these tests and hemodynamics of the patient, PE can be categorized into varying grades of clinical severity, each requiring different approaches to management to optimize outcomes.

A major goal of therapy in the management of PE is improvement of hemodynamics by reducing strain on the right ventricle. This can lead to symptom improvement, restoration of pulmonary arterial flow, decreased risk of recurrent PE, and prevention of the development of chronic thromboembolic pulmonary hypertension (CTEPH). Anticoagulation is the cornerstone of therapy for most patients with PE.[4] Patients with high-risk PE or those judged to have a high likelihood of decompensation can be considered for systemic thrombolysis or catheter-based thrombolysis. These therapies may improve symptoms and mortality[4] but place patients at elevated risks of bleeding from their systemic effects. Thrombolytic agents target fibrin via converting plasminogen to plasmin, which breaks down the fibrin,[5] resulting in partial or complete dissolution of clot, rapidly increasing the pulmonary vasculature perfusion. Advances in pharmacotherapy have led to fibrin-specific thrombolytic agents that, unlike first-generation agents (eg, streptokinase), cleave fibrin only by activating plasminogen on the surface of the clot, thus reducing its systemic effects.

RISK STRATIFICATION OF PULMONARY EMBOLISM

Historically, high-risk PE was identified through assessment of embolus burden via invasive angiography using the Miller index,[6] but its use has declined due to its invasive nature. In different studies and registries, hemodynamic instability (hypotension/circulatory shock) has been shown to be the most important determinant of short-term morbidity and mortality,[7] therefore this clinical marker helps to risk-stratify patients with PE. In an American Heart Association (AHA) scientific statement, massive PE was defined as "acute PE with sustained hypotension (systolic blood pressure <90 mm Hg for at least 15 minutes or requiring inotropic support, not due to a cause other than PE, such as arrhythmia, hypovolemia, sepsis, or left ventricular [LV] dysfunction), pulselessness, or persistent profound bradycardia (heart rate <40 bpm with signs, or symptoms of shock)."[4] These patients were considered high-risk. Patients with normal hemodynamics but objective evidence of right heart strain (via imaging or

cardiac biomarkers) were called submassive PE, which labeled a patient as intermediate risk in terms of adverse clinical outcomes. This was defined as "acute PE without systemic hypotension (systolic blood pressure ≥90 mm Hg) but with either RV [right ventricular] dysfunction or myocardial necrosis."[4] Patients without hemodynamic instability or evidence of right heart strain were considered low risk.

SELECTION OF PATIENTS FOR SYSTEMIC THROMBOLYSIS

Selecting the correct patient for systemic thrombolysis necessitates a thorough assessment of the patient's preexisting comorbidities, mode of presentation, and focused clinical examination to assess the immediate risk of hemodynamic collapse, the risk of long-term complications, and the risk of major bleeding associated with the thrombolytic agent. As described previously, high-risk PE patients warrant strong consideration of aggressive treatment options including systemic thrombolysis with a high incidence of adverse outcomes if not instituted expediently.[8] In patients who present with acute high-risk PE, the risk of mortality is high, which makes the decision for systemic thrombolysis relatively easier as compared with patients who are hemodynamically stable. The case fatality of these hemodynamically unstable patients ranges from 35% to 58%.[6,9] Therefore, benefits clearly outweigh the risk of adverse outcomes in most patients with high-risk PE who are not experiencing severe active bleeding.[10]

On the contrary, decision making in patients with intermediate-risk PE is more complex, with controversy surrounding the population-based risk of decompensation.[11] Although an analysis of the International Cooperative Pulmonary Embolism Registry in 1999 demonstrated that 15% of hemodynamically stable patients died in first 90 days of diagnosis,[7] a meta-analysis of randomized trials demonstrated only 3% short-term mortality rates in intermediate-risk patients treated with isolated anticoagulation.[10] Close monitoring of these patients is necessary with early administration of thrombolytic agent for "rescue reperfusion" if worsening hemodynamics develop. Thrombolytic therapy is not advisable in patients with low-risk PE due to a clearly unfavorable balance between improving hemodynamics and the elevated risk of intracranial and major bleeding.[12]

CLINICAL ASSESSMENT

Ideally, a prognostic model should be able to precisely identify the risk of mortality and recurrent PE in patients so that escalation of treatment can be performed when necessary. Also useful would be a risk model that predicts risks of various therapies beyond anticoagulation. Various risk prediction tools have been described in the literature with the Pulmonary Embolism Severity Index (PESI) (Table 1) being the best validated to determine short-term mortality (30-day) in patients with PE.[13] This prognostic model classifies patients from risk class I (very low risk) to class V (very high risk) based on demographics (age and sex), comorbidities (history of cancer, heart failure, chronic lung disease), and clinical findings (mentation, oxygenation, blood pressure, pulse and respiratory rate). Mortality risk range from 1% in class I patients to 24.5% in class V patients. With most patients falling in class II and class III, the negative predictive value for mortality reaches higher than 90% in low-risk patients (class I–III). Simplified PESI was also introduced, which is a modified version of previously described PESI with similar predictive precision but simpler to use. It includes age, history of heart failure or cancer, and blood pressure, pulse rate, and oxygen saturation.[14] Both prognostic models can be used to risk-stratify patients under consideration for thrombolytic therapy, but these models fail to predict the risk of adverse outcomes in these patients. In fact, there is no well-validated prediction model to assess the risk of bleeding in patients receiving thrombolysis for PE. Therefore, absolute and relative contraindications for thrombolytic therapy along with clinical judgment are the only tools available to risk-stratify for bleeding.[4,15]

BIOMARKERS AND IMAGING ASSESSMENT

Rise in cardiac biomarkers, including troponin and brain-type natriuretic peptide may represent right heart dysfunction and have been associated with an increased risk of PE-related deaths.[16–18] Chest CT scan is the gold standard imaging modality for patients who come to the emergency department with suspicion of PE. In a previous study, left and right ventricular

Table 1
Original and simplified Pulmonary Embolism Severity Index (prognostic model to predict 30-day outcomes in patients with acute pulmonary embolism)

Pulmonary Embolism Severity Index (PESI)	Simplified Pulmonary Embolism Severity Index (sPESI)
Demographics	Demographics
Age >80 y	Age >80 y
Male sex	
Comorbidities	Comorbidities
History of heart failure	History of cancer
History of cancer	History of chronic lung disease
History of chronic lung disease	
Clinical findings	Clinical findings
Tachycardia >110 beats/min	Heart rate >110/min
Systolic blood pressure <100 mm Hg	Systolic blood pressure <100 mm Hg
Respiratory rate >30/min	Arterial oxygenation saturation <90% (with or without supplemental oxygenation)
Temperature <36°C	
Altered mental status (lethargy, stupor, coma)	
Arterial oxygen saturation <90% (with or without supplemental oxygenation)	

Adapted from Aujesky D, Roy PM, Le Manach CP, et al. Validation of a model to predict adverse outcomes in patients with pulmonary embolism. Eur Heart J 2006;27(4):476–81, with permission; and Jimenez D, Aujesky D, Moores L, et al. Simplification of the pulmonary embolism severity index for prognostication in patients with acute symptomatic pulmonary embolism. Arch Intern Med 2010;170(15):1383–9; with permission.

dimensions of 431 patients with confirmed acute PE were analyzed.[19] RV enlargement, defined as RV_D/LV_D >0.9 was associated with 15.6% 30-day mortality as compared with 7.7% 30-day mortality in patients with no RV enlargement. Similarly, in another study in which 120 consecutive patients with acute PE were retrospectively studied, both the RV/LV ratio and the obstruction (Miller index) index were found to be significant risk factors for mortality at 3-month follow-up.[20] These easy-to-measure dimensions can be prognostically important in selecting patients who are at elevated risk of early deterioration.

Bedside transthoracic echocardiography can be used to detect RV dysfunction in the setting of acute PE. It can detect a wide range of imaging indicators form very nonspecific RV dilatation and hypokinesis to the very specific McConnell sign, in which the RV has a characteristic appearance of significant enlargement with free wall dysfunction and relative apical sparing.[15] In a study by Kasper and colleagues,[21] 317 patients were prospectively evaluated for right ventricular strain by echocardiography and it was found that 1-year mortality was approximately 13% in patients with RV dysfunction as compared with 1.3% in patients with no RV dysfunction. Echocardiography should be performed to further risk-stratify patients with clinical evidence of RV failure, elevated cardiac enzymes, or in clinical decompensation. All these modalities can be helpful in not only classifying these patients as intermediate or high risk, but also to segregate patients with high likelihood of early deterioration so that systemic thrombolysis can be used.[22]

Summarizing the patient selection criteria for systemic thrombolysis, it is clear that the clinical judgment to use a thrombolytic agent in addition to anticoagulation in a patient with acute PE necessitates an individualized assessment of the benefits[23] of improving morbidity and mortality versus the risk of major bleeding.

EVIDENCE OF IMPROVEMENT IN CLINICAL OUTCOMES WITH THROMBOLYSIS IN PATIENTS WITH HIGH-RISK PULMONARY EMBOLISM

It has been more than 4 decades since the first use of systemic thrombolysis by Miller and colleagues[6] in 1971 in patients with acute PE. Early randomized controlled trials failed to show any evidence of mortality benefit with the use of thrombolytic agents in comparison with intravenous heparin therapy in patients with PE, although promising results were seen with regard to clot resolution and improving the hemodynamics of patients. The role of thrombolytic therapy in patients with high-risk PE resulting in hemodynamic instability and cardiogenic shock has not been well studied in randomized clinical trials (RCTs) due to a perceived lack of equipoise for randomization in this population given the high rates of short-term mortality with conservative therapies. In the early 1990s, Jerjes-Sanchez and colleagues[24] randomized 8 patients with high-risk PE to receive either heparin with streptokinase or isolated heparin. All 4 patients who received streptokinase improved quickly and survived without any major side effects at 2 years of follow-up. On the contrary, all 4 patients died in the heparin group from RV failure due to massive PE (confirmed on autopsy). This is the main published data that has led to the consensus in guidelines that reperfusion with systemic thrombolysis (in the absence of absolute contraindications) is indicated in patients who present with high-risk PE.[4,15] In patients with relative and absolute contraindications to the use of systemic thrombolysis (**Table 2**), other therapies, including catheter-based therapies, should be considered.[25]

EVIDENCE OF BENEFITS IN PATIENTS WITH INTERMEDIATE-RISK PULMONARY EMBOLISM

Evidence of beneficial effects of systemic thrombolysis in patient with intermediate-risk PE has been a topic rife with controversy. Conflicting results from RCTs, registries, and meta-analyses have led to less robust guidelines to manage these apparently stable patients. Traditionally, intravenous anticoagulation with heparin has been considered sufficient to resolve the clot and prevent further morbidity, but some studies raise concerns that a portion of these patients with RV dysfunction may be at intermediate risk for early decompensation.[15,26] As mentioned previously, prognostic models can be useful for supplementing clinical judgment in the management of patients with PE with different risks of decompensation.[27–29] Importantly, unlike in the setting of high-risk PE, there is also a fairly robust evidence base to assist in our decision making.

In 2002, Konstantinides and colleagues[9] published data from an RCT that randomized 256 patients to alteplase versus conservative therapy for intermediate-risk PE. The group receiving

Table 2
Contraindications to systemic thrombolysis in patients with acute pulmonary embolism

Absolute Contraindications	Relative Contraindications
• Prior intracranial hemorrhage	• History of chronic severe uncontrolled hypertension
• Known structural cerebral lesion	• Severe uncontrolled hypertension (systolic >180 mm Hg or diastolic >110 mm Hg
• Known malignant intracranial neoplasm	• History of ischemic cerebrovascular accident >3 mo
• Ischemic stroke within 3 mo	• Trauma or prolonged cardiopulmonary resuscitation >10 min
• Suspected aortic dissection	• Major surgery within 3 wk
• Active bleeding (excluding menses)	• Recent internal bleed (2–4 wk)
• Significant closed-head or face trauma within 3 mo	• Pregnancy, active peptic ulcer, pericarditis, age >75 y, diabetic retinopathy, recent invasive procedure, current anticoagulant use

Up to two-thirds of patients with acute PE do not receive thrombolytic therapy due to contraindications.

Adapted from Konstantinides SV, Torbicki A, Agnelli G, et al. 2014 ESC guidelines on the diagnosis and management of acute pulmonary embolism. Eur Heart J 2014;35(43):3033–69, 3069a–k; with permission.

alteplase, with a background of anticoagulation therapy, as initial therapy for submassive PE showed improved 30-day event-free survival as compared with heparin plus placebo. This was largely driven by a reduction in need for escalation of therapy (ie, initiation of pressors or resuscitation from cardiac arrest) in the thrombolytic arm. This study opened the discussion for the intermediate-risk PE which at that time was recommended only for high-risk PE. Subsequently, the international PEITHO (Pulmonary Embolism Thrombolysis) trial[30] randomized 1006 patients with a similar design. Single intravenous bolus of tenecteplase plus heparin showed benefits in prevention of hemodynamic decompensation when compared with placebo plus heparin in patients with intermediate-risk PE. In the tenecteplase group, although the primary outcome of all-cause death or hemodynamic decompensation/collapse within 7 days occurred significantly less

often than in the group receiving heparin alone, a concerning trend toward increased intracranial bleeding and major nonintracranial bleeding was seen.[30] Over the past decade, many additional smaller RCTs have been performed with variable results. A systematic review and meta-analysis by Chatterjee and colleagues[10] attempted to reconcile these data through analysis of the mortality, major bleeding, and intracranial hemorrhage (ICH) rates in the 8 RCTs that have studied intermediate-risk PE. The investigators concluded that although there was potential mortality benefit with thrombolytic therapy among the population of patients with intermediate-risk PE in contemporary clinical practice, this comes at the expense of increased major bleeding events and ICH. Specifically the number needed to treat (NNT) to prevent 1 death was 59, and the NNT to prevent a recurrent PE event was 54. The benefit was offset by the risk of major bleeds (number needed to harm [NNH]) of 18, with an NNH for ICH of 78. Although varying doses and types of thrombolytic agents were used in different studies, this was the first meta-analysis with sufficient statistical power to show mortality benefit. Also of significance is that the short-term mortality rate of patients treated only with anticoagulation in this pooled analysis was 3.89% (41 deaths of 1054 patients with PE treated with anticoagulation), with the rate in intermediate-risk patients less than 3%. Although clinical trial populations are not totally representative of those treated in general clinical care, this calls into question the mortality range of 3% to 15% range specified for patients with intermediate-risk PE in the current AHA guidelines[26] (**Table 3**). The low baseline mortality rate makes the threshold high for escalating therapy beyond anticoagulants for the prevention of acute mortality. Another postulated reason for administering thrombolytic therapy is the prevention of CTEPH. However, longer-term follow-up from the PEITHO trial suggested therapeutic equivalence with thrombolytics compared with anticoagulation alone for the prevention of subsequent CTEPH after acute PE.[31]

In view of these equivocal data, it is prudent to risk-stratify these patients before deciding to give thrombolytic agents in these stable patients. Rigorously examining the benefits versus risks using clinical judgment, prognostic models and consideration of other possible treatment options should be performed in patients who are intermediate risk. The evidence base at present does not support thrombolytic therapy in all patients with intermediate-risk PE. However, acknowledging the possibility of benefit in

Table 3
Latest recommendations for systemic thrombolysis in patients with acute massive and submassive pulmonary embolism (PE)

Society	Entity	Recommendations
American College of Chest Physicians,[25] 2016	Massive PE with low bleeding risk	Grade 2B
	Submassive PE	Grade 1B
	Patients with submassive PE who deteriorate (not developed hypotension yet) and low bleeding risk	Grade 2C
American Heart Association,[26] 2011	Massive PE	Class IIa, Level of Evidence B
	Submassive PE with evidence of adverse prognosis and low bleeding risk	Class IIb, Level of Evidence C
	Submassive PE	Class III; Level of Evidence B
European Society of Cardiology,[15] 2014	Massive PE	Class I; Level of Evidence B
	Submassive PE	Class III, Level of Evidence B

some patients,[10] ongoing research efforts should try to identify those most likely to benefit with minimal trade-off of risk.

EVIDENCE OF BENEFITS OF SYSTEMIC THROMBOLYSIS IN LOW-RISK PULMONARY EMBOLISM

Patients with neither hemodynamic compromise nor any evidence of RV dysfunction or myocardial injury are considered low risk, and use of systemic thrombolysis is not recommended (Grade III, level of evidence B).[26] These patients have short-term mortality rates of 1% or less from the acute PE, so any potential benefits are outweighed by the bleeding risks of thrombolysis. Isolated anticoagulation remains the mainstay of treatment in these patients.

ASSESSMENT OF BLEEDING RISK

One of the determinants of outcomes with thrombolytic use especially in patients with intermediate-risk PE is a judicious assessment of bleeding risk, especially of intracranial bleeds. Conventional risk scores used to assess bleeding risk with use of anticoagulants in different populations like HASBLED and ATRIA have poor predictive ability to identify potential for major bleeding with PE.[32] Ongoing research efforts are directed toward developing risk assessment tools for predicting the risk of major bleeding and intracranial hemorrhage,[33] although these efforts have been hindered by the inadequacy of currently available population-based datasets for PE. The most consistent marker of risk for bleeding with systemic thrombolysis among patients with PE is

increasing age. Observational data have demonstrated significantly increased risks with age older than 65, whereas the PEITHO trial identified most ICH events occurring in patients older than 75.[30,33]

NEW CATHETER-BASED TREATMENT OPTIONS

Interestingly, the concept of using catheter-based techniques to manage patients with PE has roots that predate the initial consideration of systemic thrombolysis in these patients. The Food and Drug Administration approved deployment of Greenfield suction catheters in 1969 to remove thrombus from the pulmonary vasculature. Currently, many catheter-mediated techniques have been used in the pulmonary arteries.[34–41] Extensive details regarding these techniques are available in Bedros Taslakian and Akhilesh K. Sista's article, "Catheter Directed Therapy for Pulmonary Embolism: Patient Selection and Technical Considerations" and Wissam A Jaber and colleagues' article, "Catheter-Based Embolectomy for Acute Pulmonary Embolism: Devices, Technical Considerations, Risks & Benefits," elsewhere in this issue.

MANAGEMENT PROTOCOLS

In the recent PEITHO trial,[30] the patients randomized to receive fibrinolytics received a single weight-based intravenous bolus (given over a period of 5–10 seconds) of the fibrinolytic agent tenecteplase. The dose ranged from 30 mg to 50 mg, depending on body weight. Another trial[23] assessed low-dose thrombolytics for reduction of recurrent PE or subsequent development of pulmonary hypertension. Alteplase 0.5 mg/kg (maximum 50 mg), given as a 10-mg bolus followed by the remainder over 2 hours, was associated with a reduction in pulmonary hypertension (16% vs 57%) as well as the composite outcome of pulmonary hypertension or recurrent PE (16% vs 63%). European Society of Cardiology (ESC) has published "approved" thrombolytic regimens for pulmonary embolism[15]: streptokinase 250,000 IU as a loading dose over 30 minutes, followed by 100,000 IU/h over 12 to 24 hours, accelerated regimen:

1.5 million IU over 2 hours; urokinase 4400 IU/kg as a loading dose over 10 minutes, followed by 4400 IU/kg per hour over 12 to 24 hours, accelerated regimen 3 million IU over 2 hours; alteplase 100 mg over 2 hours or 0.6 mg/kg over 15 minutes (maximum dose 50 mg). A definitive trial looking at comparisons of different dosing regimens for intravenous (IV) thrombolysis in acute PE has not been performed to date.

The following is a "real-life" protocol for systemic thrombolysis followed by the PE response team at the Hospital of the University of Pennsylvania:

Procedures before/ after alteplase	• If possible and indicated, place nasogastric tubes, indwelling bladder catheters, intra-arterial lines, or intravenous lines before administration of systemic alteplase. • If unable to perform before therapy, delay placement of nasogastric tubes, indwelling bladder catheters, intra-arterial pressure catheters, or intravenous lines for 24 hours if possible.
Alteplase dosing	Massive (or submassive) PE: • 100-mg IV infusion over 2 h for most patients. • In patients at high risk of bleeding, relative contraindications (see Table 1), age >65 y, weight <65 kg, body mass index <25 kg/m², a dose of 50-mg IV infusion over 1 h may be considered (or recommended by the PERT attending). Cardiac arrest: • Registered nurse (RN) may administer (physician/advanced practitioner can give if they prefer). • 50-mg IV over 2–5 min. • Once alteplase is given for cardiac arrest, high-quality cardiopulmonary resuscitation (CPR) should be continued at least 15 min after the dose to allow drug to circulate. CPR should be continued while alteplase is being administered. ○ If no return of spontaneous circulation 15 min after alteplase bolus: can consider a second 50 mg IV over 2–5 min. ○ If return of spontaneous circulation after alteplase 50-mg bolus: give remaining 50-mg IV infusion over 1 h.
Concomitant anticoagulation	• IV unfractionated heparin (UFH) in full therapeutic doses is the preferred anticoagulant for those receiving alteplase for PE before alteplase infusion. • While considering/preparing alteplase, initiate UFH treatment with a bolus as endorsed by the Recommended Protocols for Initiation and Maintenance for Heparin Therapy and Prophylaxis for Non-Neonates on the PennMedicine Formulary. • Once the decision to give alteplase is made, alteplase should be given as soon as possible. Suspend IV UFH treatment immediately before the initiation of alteplase infusion and throughout infusion. • When the alteplase infusion is complete, check an aPTT immediately and restart UFH without a bolus at the previous infusion rate if aPTT <80 s. • If a patient received a therapeutic dose of enoxaparin before alteplase, start the UFH infusion 12 h after the last dose of low-molecular weight heparin (LMWH) (24 h if given dalteparin/fondaparinux), provided the patient does not have new renal dysfunction, and did not receive a 1.5-mg/kg enoxaparin dose. If either of the latter two occur, please contact a critical care clinical pharmacy specialist for guidance. • After 48–72 h of stability, the patient may be transitioned to a LMWH, warfarin, or a novel oral anticoagulant as clinically indicated.

(continued on next page)

Administration	A dedicated IV line is required; may be given peripherally 100-mg or 50-mg alteplase dose slow infusion (RN): • Must be given via IV infusion pump. • Can be found in library under alteplase → pulmonary embolism. • VTBI entered should be 100 mL (or 50 mL for 50-mg dose). • Rate of infusion will be 50 mL/h. • When there is no alteplase left in the vial but drug left in the drip chamber, a 0.9% sodium chloride IV bag (100 mL or 250 mL as available on the unit) should be spiked and attached to the IV tubing where the empty vial was to continue to run at the same rate (50 mL/h) to complete the 2 (or 1 as stated based on dose above) -hour infusion time. No need for further modifications to IV.
Administration (continued)	Infusion pump, when pump is finished infusing, discard the remainder of the sodium chloride bag. This will ensure patient receives the entire dose ordered at correct rate (approximate IV tubing space is approximately 25–28 mL). 50-mg bolus–cardiac arrest dose (RN or physician/advanced practitioner): • RN may administer (physician/advanced practitioner may give if they prefer) IV over 2–5 min (rate of administration may be prolonged in patients with smaller-gauge IV catheters). • When RN administers medication, ordering provider must remain at bedside during administration.

Monitoring/ intensive care unit (ICU) care until 24 h after alteplase administration	Alteplase therapy can be initiated on all floors. If alteplase is initiated on the floor, patients should be transferred to an ICU as soon as possible, as critical care nursing and an ICU bed are required. Patients should remain in the ICU for the duration of the alteplase infusion and for at least 24 h after completion of the alteplase infusion.
	Obtain baseline assessment of hemodynamics and laboratory data.
	Perform neurologic assessments (add neuro parameter to the vital signs flowsheet)
	• Every 15 min during the infusion, then
	• Every 30 min thereafter for the next 6 h, then
	• Hourly until 24 h after treatment
	Blood pressure (BP) monitoring
	• Every 15 min for the first 2 h, then
	• Every 30 min for the next 6 h, then
	  ○ Hourly until 24 h after treatment
	  ○ BP must be maintained at or below 180/105 mm Hg for 24 h
	  ○ Increase the frequency (per primary team) if a systolic BP is >180 mm Hg or if a diastolic BP is >105 mm Hg; administer antihypertensive medications to maintain BP at or below these levels.
	Bleeding precautions
	  ○ Check puncture sites for hematomas.
	  ○ Apply digital pressure or pressure dressing to active compressible bleeding sites.
	  ○ Visual inspection of urine, stool, and emesis for blood.
	  ○ Monitor patient for evidence of gingival bleeding.

Management of common adverse events	Bleeding • If serious bleeding occurs during or after the alteplase infusion, alteplase should be discontinued immediately with a consideration of suspending UFH as well. If RN discovers, immediately notify covering provider. Allergic reactions • Orolingual angioedema has been observed in up to 5% of patients who receive alteplase. If angioedema develops, stop infusion and treat with supportive therapy (airway management, histamine antagonists, steroids).

Abbreviations: aPTT, activated partial thromboplastin time; PERT, pulmonary embolism response team; VTBI, volume to be infused.

LATEST GUIDELINES

Summary recommendations: Available data suggest that the following patients may derive significant benefits with thrombolytic administration potentially justifying the substantial risks of bleeding:

1. Patients with high-risk PE who are not experiencing acute cardiovascular collapse (ie, may need mechanical support first) and no bleeding contraindication.
2. High-risk patients experiencing acute cardiovascular collapse in a setting in which mechanical circulatory support is not immediately available.
3. Highest end of intermediate-risk patients (ie, those with characteristics such as high PESI score, significant tachycardia, significant hypoxemia, or dramatically reduced functional capacity even after an initial 24 to 48 hours of anticoagulation therapy) and no bleeding contraindications.

In patients in the previous 2 categories with a higher bleeding risk, catheter-directed therapies may be an appropriate option.

SUMMARY

Systemic thrombolysis has been proven to be the preferred initial therapy for patients who are hemodynamically unstable, and consideration can be given to patients who are stable but are at increased risk of clinical deterioration. The associated risks of major bleeding and ICH are significantly elevated with thrombolytic therapy, although there may be reduced harm in patients younger than 65 years. Optimal and pragmatic selection of patients to receive thrombolytic agents can be challenging, and should involve a multidisciplinary approach.

REFERENCES

1. Anderson FA Jr, Wheeler HB, Goldberg RJ, et al. A population-based perspective of the hospital incidence and case-fatality rates of deep vein thrombosis and pulmonary embolism. The Worcester DVT Study. Arch Intern Med 1991; 151(5):933–8.
2. Kubista E. Breast cancer: figures and facts. Wien Med Wochenschr 2001;151(21–23):548–51 [in German].
3. Kniffin WD Jr, Baron JA, Barrett J, et al. The epidemiology of diagnosed pulmonary embolism and deep venous thrombosis in the elderly. Arch Intern Med 1994;154(8):861–6.
4. Kearon C, Akl EA, Comerota AJ, et al. Antithrombotic therapy for VTE disease: Antithrombotic Therapy and Prevention of Thrombosis, 9th ed: American College of Chest Physicians Evidence-Based Clinical Practice Guidelines. Chest 2012; 141(2 Suppl):e419S–496.
5. Weinberg I, Jaff MR. Accelerated thrombolysis for pulmonary embolism: will clinical benefit be ULTI-MAtely realized? Circulation 2014;129(4):420–1.
6. Miller GA, Sutton GC, Kerr IH, et al. Comparison of streptokinase and heparin in treatment of isolated acute massive pulmonary embolism. Br Med J 1971;2(5763):681–4.
7. Goldhaber SZ, Visani L, De Rosa M. Acute pulmonary embolism: clinical outcomes in the International Cooperative Pulmonary Embolism Registry (ICOPER). Lancet 1999;353(9162):1386–9.
8. Marti C, John G, Konstantinides S, et al. Systemic thrombolytic therapy for acute pulmonary embolism: a systematic review and meta-analysis. Eur Heart J 2015;36(10):605–14.
9. Konstantinides S, Geibel A, Heusel G, et al. Heparin plus alteplase compared with heparin alone in patients with submassive pulmonary embolism. N Engl J Med 2002;347(15):1143–50.
10. Chatterjee S, Chakraborty A, Weinberg I, et al. Thrombolysis for pulmonary embolism and risk of all-cause mortality, major bleeding, and intracranial hemorrhage: a meta-analysis. JAMA 2014;311(23): 2414–21.
11. Vedantham S, Piazza G, Sista AK, et al. Guidance for the use of thrombolytic therapy for the treatment of venous thromboembolism. J Thromb Thrombolysis 2016;41(1):68–80.
12. Meyer G, Vieillard-Baron A, Planquette B. Recent advances in the management of pulmonary embolism: focus on the critically ill patients. Ann Intensive Care 2016;6(1):19.
13. Aujesky D, Roy PM, Le Manach CP, et al. Validation of a model to predict adverse outcomes in patients with pulmonary embolism. Eur Heart J 2006;27(4): 476–81.
14. Jimenez D, Aujesky D, Moores L, et al. Simplification of the pulmonary embolism severity index for prognostication in patients with acute symptomatic pulmonary embolism. Arch Intern Med 2010; 170(15):1383–9.
15. Konstantinides SV, Torbicki A, Agnelli G, et al. 2014 ESC guidelines on the diagnosis and management of acute pulmonary embolism. Eur Heart J 2014; 35(43):3033–69, 3069a–k.
16. Piazza G, Goldhaber SZ. Management of submassive pulmonary embolism. Circulation 2010; 122(11):1124–9.
17. Stein PD, Matta F, Janjua M, et al. Outcome in stable patients with acute pulmonary embolism who had right ventricular enlargement and/or elevated

levels of troponin I. Am J Cardiol 2010;106(4): 558–63.

18. Giannitsis E, Muller-Bardorff M, Kurowski V, et al. Independent prognostic value of cardiac troponin T in patients with confirmed pulmonary embolism. Circulation 2000;102(2):211–7.

19. Schoepf UJ, Kucher N, Kipfmueller F, et al. Right ventricular enlargement on chest computed tomography: a predictor of early death in acute pulmonary embolism. Circulation 2004;110(20):3276–80.

20. van der Meer RW, Pattynama PM, van Strijen MJ, et al. Right ventricular dysfunction and pulmonary obstruction index at helical CT: prediction of clinical outcome during 3-month follow-up in patients with acute pulmonary embolism. Radiology 2005; 235(3):798–803.

21. Kasper W, Konstantinides S, Geibel A, et al. Prognostic significance of right ventricular afterload stress detected by echocardiography in patients with clinically suspected pulmonary embolism. Heart 1997;77(4):346–9.

22. Terrin M, Goldhaber SZ, Thompson B. Selection of patients with acute pulmonary embolism for thrombolytic therapy. Thrombolysis in pulmonary embolism (TIPE) patient survey. The TIPE Investigators. Chest 1989;95(5 Suppl):279s–81s.

23. Sharifi M, Bay C, Skrocki L, et al. Moderate pulmonary embolism treated with thrombolysis (from the "MOPETT" Trial). Am J Cardiol 2013;111(2):273–7.

24. Jerjes-Sanchez C, Ramirez-Rivera A, de Lourdes Garcia M, et al. Streptokinase and heparin versus heparin alone in massive pulmonary embolism: a randomized controlled trial. J Thromb Thrombolysis 1995;2(3):227–9.

25. Kearon C, Akl EA, Ornelas J, et al. Antithrombotic Therapy for VTE Disease: CHEST Guideline and Expert Panel Report. Chest 2016;149(2):315–52.

26. Jaff MR, McMurtry MS, Archer SL, et al. Management of massive and submassive pulmonary embolism, iliofemoral deep vein thrombosis, and chronic thromboembolic pulmonary hypertension: a scientific statement from the American Heart Association. Circulation 2011;123(16):1788–830.

27. Vanni S, Nazerian P, Pepe G, et al. Comparison of two prognostic models for acute pulmonary embolism: clinical vs. right ventricular dysfunction-guided approach. J Thromb Haemost 2011;9(10):1916–23.

28. Becattini C, Agnelli G, Salvi A, et al. Bolus tenecteplase for right ventricle dysfunction in hemodynamically stable patients with pulmonary embolism. Thromb Res 2010;125(3):e82–6.

29. Kline JA, Nordenholz KE, Courtney DM, et al. Treatment of submassive pulmonary embolism with tenecteplase or placebo: cardiopulmonary outcomes at 3 months: multicenter double-blind, placebo-controlled randomized trial. J Thromb Haemost 2014;12(4):459–68.

30. Meyer G, Vicaut E, Danays T, et al. Fibrinolysis for patients with intermediate-risk pulmonary embolism. N Engl J Med 2014;370(15):1402–11.

31. Konstantinides SV, Vicaut E, Danays T, et al. Impact of thrombolytic therapy on the long-term outcome of intermediate-risk pulmonary embolism. J Am Coll Cardiol 2017 Mar 28;69(12):1536–44.

32. Chatterjee S, Lip GY, Giri J. HAS-BLED versus ATRIA risk scores for intracranial hemorrhage in patients receiving thrombolytics for pulmonary embolism. J Am Coll Cardiol 2016;67(24):2904–5.

33. Chatterjee S, Weinberg I, Yeh RW, et al. Risk factors for intracranial haemorrhage in patients with pulmonary embolism treated with thrombolytic therapy. Development of the PE-CH Score. Thromb Haemost 2017;117(2):246–51.

34. Dumantepe M, Teymen B, Akturk U, et al. Efficacy of rotational thrombectomy on the mortality of patients with massive and submassive pulmonary embolism. J Card Surg 2015;30(4):324–32.

35. Jaber WA, Fong PP, Weisz G, et al. Acute pulmonary embolism: with an emphasis on an interventional approach. J Am Coll Cardiol 2016;67(8): 991–1002.

36. Kuo WT, Banerjee A, Kim PS, et al. Pulmonary Embolism Response to Fragmentation, Embolectomy, and Catheter Thrombolysis (PERFECT): initial results from a prospective multicenter registry. Chest 2015;148(3):667–73.

37. Piazza G, Hohlfelder B, Jaff MR, et al. A prospective, single-arm, multicenter trial of ultrasound-facilitated, catheter-directed, low-dose fibrinolysis for acute massive and submassive pulmonary embolism: the SEATTLE II Study. JACC Cardiovasc Interv 2015;8(10):1382–92.

38. Kuo WT, Gould MK, Louie JD, et al. Catheter-directed therapy for the treatment of massive pulmonary embolism: systematic review and meta-analysis of modern techniques. J Vasc Interv Radiol 2009;20(11):1431–40.

39. Kucher N, Boekstegers P, Muller OJ, et al. Randomized, controlled trial of ultrasound-assisted catheter-directed thrombolysis for acute intermediate-risk pulmonary embolism. Circulation 2014;129(4):479–86.

40. Jickling GC, Zhan X, Ander BP, et al. Genome response to tissue plasminogen activator in experimental ischemic stroke. BMC Genomics 2010;11:254.

41. Jazi SM, Nazary IA, Behjati M. Response to thrombolytic agents in acute myocardial infarction in opium abusers versus non-abusers. J Res Pharm Pract 2012;1(1):34–6.

Catheter-Directed Therapy for Pulmonary Embolism
Patient Selection and Technical Considerations

Bedros Taslakian, MD[a], Akhilesh K. Sista, MD[b],*

KEYWORDS

- Pulmonary embolism • Thrombolysis • Catheter-directed therapy
- Catheter-directed thrombolysis

KEY POINTS

- Acute pulmonary embolism (PE) remains a significant cause of cardiovascular morbidity and mortality worldwide. Immediate recognition, triaging, and treatment of patients presenting with acute PE is imperative.
- The mainstay of acute PE treatment is anticoagulation; low-risk PE can be treated with anticoagulation alone and has an excellent prognosis. However, given the high mortality associated with high-risk PE, more aggressive therapy options have been suggested. The optimal strategy for intermediate-risk PE, beyond anticoagulation, is unknown and still controversial.
- High-risk or massive PE carries a significant mortality, and patients may die within an hour of presentation; therefore, societal guidelines agree on treatment escalation with primary reperfusion. Emerging patterns of care in this population include hemodynamic stabilization with mechanical hemodynamic support as a bridge to decision on definitive therapy.
- Catheter-directed therapy is an adjunct or alternative to systemic thrombolysis and surgical thromboembolectomy in patients with high-risk PE.
- The routine use of catheter-directed thrombolysis for intermediate-risk PE cannot be recommended based on current data. A rigorous, randomized trial is needed to define risks and benefits of catheter-directed thrombolysis in the intermediate-risk PE population.

INTRODUCTION

Acute pulmonary embolism (PE) is the third leading cause of death among hospitalized patients.[1,2] Approximately 100,000 to 180,000 patients with PE die annually in the United States.[3–5] In those who survive the initial insult, PE can lead to long-term disability, such as chronic thromboembolic pulmonary hypertension, persistent right ventricular (RV) dysfunction, impaired functional status, diminished exercise capacity, and reduced quality of life.[6–9] Successful management of acute PE requires swift recognition, prompt risk stratification, and decisive early treatment. Although patients with low-risk PE have an excellent

---

Conflict of Interest: B. Taslakian reports no conflict of interest. A.K. Sista received a research grant from Penumbra, Inc, administered through the NYU Department of Radiology.

[a] Vascular and Interventional Radiology, Department of Radiology, NYU Langone Medical Center, 550 First Avenue, 2nd Floor (VIR Section), New York, NY 10016, USA; [b] Vascular and Interventional Radiology, Department of Radiology, NYU Langone Medical Center, 660 First Avenue, 3rd Floor, New York, NY 10016, USA
* Corresponding author.
E-mail address: Akhilesh.Sista@nyumc.org

Intervent Cardiol Clin 7 (2018) 81–90
http://dx.doi.org/10.1016/j.iccl.2017.08.002
2211-7458/18/© 2017 Elsevier Inc. All rights reserved.

prognosis (<1% mortality) and are adequately treated with therapeutic doses of anticoagulation alone, patients with high-risk or intermediate-risk PE have 20% to 50% and 3% to 9% short-term mortalities, respectively.[10,11] Most of the deaths in hemodynamically unstable patients occur within the first hour of presentation.[12] The poor outcomes associated with high-risk and intermediate-risk PE despite anticoagulation have prompted some physicians to consider therapeutic escalation through systemic thrombolysis, catheter-directed therapy, and/or surgical embolectomy.

This article focuses on the use of catheter-directed therapy for severe acute PE. Selection criteria, societal guidelines, and controversies in the literature are reviewed. A systematic approach to the periprocedural period is provided.

PULMONARY EMBOLISM RISK STRATIFICATION

Once PE is diagnosed, immediate risk stratification allows rapid triaging. Given the complexity of management and various treatment options for patients with severe PE, multidisciplinary PE response teams have emerged.[13,14] The main role of a PE response team is to rapidly assess and stratify patients presenting with acute severe PE. By reviewing the patient's clinical status, comorbidities, imaging and biomarker results, bleeding risk, and hemodynamics, the team can select the patients who may benefit from treatment escalation.

All major guideline committees, including the American College of Chest Physicians (ACCP), the American Heart Association (AHA), and the European Society of Cardiology (ESC), have adopted a risk-based prognostic stratification strategy to guide the management of acute PE.[5,11,15,16] Acute PE was classified by the AHA into 3 major categories: massive, submassive, and low risk.[11] In 2014, The ESC proposed an alternative model for risk stratification. The ESC's PE categories include high-risk, intermediate-risk, and low-risk PE.[5] The ESC acknowledges the complexity of risk stratification and management of the intermediate-risk PE (submassive) category, which encompasses a broad range of presentations, and further stratifies this group into high-risk and low-risk intermediate PE. Also, the ESC guidelines recognize the role of other clinical parameters and include the pulmonary embolism severity index (PESI) and its simplified version (simplified PESI [sPESI]) as tools to assess patient mortality risk.

PULMONARY EMBOLISM MANAGEMENT

In patients with acute PE, regardless of its severity, parenteral anticoagulation is recommended unless contraindicated. Although anticoagulants do not lyse the clot, they can allow the natural thrombolytic system to function unopposed, ultimately decreasing the thromboembolic burden.[1] Although low-risk PE can be adequately treated with anticoagulation alone and has an excellent prognosis, guidelines suggest primary reperfusion, particularly with systemic thrombolysis for high-risk PE (ie, full-dose tissue plasminogen activator [tPA]).[5,11,15,16] The currently approved protocol for systemic thrombolysis in patients with acute high-risk PE is 100 mg of tPA (alteplase; Genentech, South San Francisco, CA) infused intravenously (IV) over a period of 2 hours.[11] In patients with contraindications to thrombolysis, severe hemodynamic collapse that is likely to cause death before full-dose IV tPA infusion can take effect, and in whom systemic thrombolysis fails to improve hemodynamic status, societal guidelines suggest, if appropriate expertise and resources are available, considering surgical embolectomy or percutaneous catheter-directed therapy.[5,11,15,16] Recent retrospective cohort studies showed a much lower mortality than historical rates with contemporary surgical embolectomy.[17–19] Surgical embolectomy can also be a viable option in special circumstances, including RV clot in transit or a patent foramen ovale.[11,15] In a meta-analysis of 594 patients with acute high-risk PE treated with catheter-directed therapy (catheter-directed mechanical fragmentation, aspiration of emboli, and/or intraclot thrombolytic injection), the clinical success rate (defined as the stabilization of hemodynamics, survival to hospital discharge, and resolution of hypoxia) was 86.5% and the rate of major procedural complications was 2.4%.[20] Although these statistics are encouraging, the meta-analysis had 2 important limitations: (1) no randomized trials were included, and (2) the majority of trials were retrospective with a small number of patients. In this study, 96% of patients received catheter-directed therapy as the first adjunct to anticoagulation with no previous systemic tPA infusion, and 33% of cases were performed with stand-alone mechanical thrombectomy (ie, received no thrombolytic during catheter-directed therapy).[20] In select patients who are in extremis from high-risk PE and have no contraindication to thrombolysis, it may be desirable to initiate emergent systemic thrombolysis while simultaneously activating the interventional team to perform catheter-directed therapy and mechanically debulk the clot, allowing rapid pulmonary arterial blood restoration and reduction of the dose of IV tPA.[21]

In contrast, there is uncertainty regarding the optimal therapy for patients with intermediate-risk PE, which has a higher rate of clinical deterioration and mortality than low-risk PE but a lower mortality than high-risk PE. One of the key unanswered questions is whether patients with intermediate-risk PE should be routinely considered for therapeutic escalation beyond anticoagulation.[22] Systemic thrombolysis in particular has been extensively studied in acute intermediate-risk PE. Meta-analysis data show a small mortality benefit and a lower rate of clinical deterioration at the cost of significantly higher major and intracranial bleeding rates.[23,24] The recent Pulmonary Embolism Thrombolysis (PEITHO) study randomly assigned 1005 anticoagulated patients with intermediate-risk PE to bolus tenecteplase or placebo.[25] The primary outcome (ie, death or hemodynamic decompensation at 7 days of randomization) occurred significantly more often in the placebo group, although all-cause mortality at 30 days was not significantly different. However, major and intracranial bleeding occurred significantly more often in the tenecteplase group.

Catheter directed thrombolysis (CDT) has garnered interest because of the limitations of both anticoagulation and systemic thrombolysis in the treatment of intermediate-risk PE group. However, the level of evidence supporting its efficacy and safety is much lower than that of systemic thrombolysis.[22] There are 3 prospective clinical trials examining CDT in the setting of intermediate-risk and high-risk PE: Ultrasound Accelerated Thrombolysis of Pulmonary Embolism (ULTIMA),[26] SEATTLE II,[27] and Pulmonary Embolism Response to Fragmentation, Embolectomy, and Catheter Thrombolysis (PERFECT).[28] These studies have shown a statistically significant reduction in pulmonary artery pressures (PAPs) and improvement in RV function and pulmonary blood flow in patients undergoing CDT.[26–28] Importantly, similar improvements in surrogate end points have been seen with trials and observational studies of systemic thrombolysis.[29]

ULTIMA, which included 59 patients, was the only randomized trial comparing CDT with anticoagulation. SEATTLE II was a single-arm study of CDT and had a larger sample size of 150 patients, 119 of whom had intermediate-risk PE. There were no intracranial or fatal bleeding events in 178 patients with intermediate-risk PE

evaluated in the ULTIMA and SEATTLE II studies; 10% of patients had major bleeding complications in SEATTLE II and none in ULTIMA.[26,27] The PERFECT registry, which also lacked a control arm, included 101 patients with high-risk and intermediate-risk PE. There were no major or intracranial bleeds with CDT.[28] However, these studies are preliminary and their data do not justify routine use of CDT for intermediate-risk PE. The studies did not robustly evaluate clinically relevant short-term and long-term outcomes. Because of the increased risk of major and intracranial bleeding in patients treated with systemic thrombolysis[23–25] and the paucity of strong data on CDT's effectiveness and safety in the treatment of intermediate-risk PE, anticoagulation alone is still considered the standard of care for most patients with intermediate-risk PE based on current evidence.[5,11,15,16] In addition, no randomized trial has compared systemic administration of thrombolytics with CDT.

CATHETER-DIRECTED THERAPY FOR SEVERE PULMONARY EMBOLISM

Several catheter-based techniques exist for rapid removal of thrombus from the pulmonary arteries (PAs) to immediately restore blood flow to the pulmonary circulation, with subsequent improvement in the RV strain, hemodynamic status, and oxygenation.[28,30] The choice of procedure and tools differs based on the severity of the PE and estimated bleeding risk.

For treatment of high-risk PE, the goal is rapid central clot removal to relieve life-threatening RV strain and immediately improve pulmonary perfusion. Depending on bleeding risk, pharmacomechanical thrombolysis or stand-alone catheter-directed mechanical thrombectomy can be performed. Percutaneous mechanical thrombectomy in patients with high risk of bleeding achieves central thrombus removal without fibrinolytic drug infusion. Details of various embolus removal techniques are discussed in Wissam A. Jaber and Michael C. McDaniel's article, "Catheter-Based Embolectomy for Acute Pulmonary Embolism: Devices, Technical Considerations, Risks & Benefits," in this issue. Pharmacomechanical thrombolysis is performed by catheter-directed injection of a thrombolytic drug in conjunction with mechanical clot fragmentation, aspiration, and/or maceration to further promote clot disaggregation by exposing a greater surface area of thrombus to endogenous and/or locally infused fibrinolytics. Complete thrombus removal is not the goal of these percutaneous methods; instead, downstaging from high-risk to intermediate-risk PE suffices.

In intermediate-risk PE, mechanical debulking is unproved and is potentially risky, because clot fragmentation may lead to distal embolization resulting in acute increase of PA resistance and RV afterload.[21,30] The goal for CDT is to achieve similar efficacy to systemic thrombolysis and potentially decrease the rate of major and intra-cranial bleeding by delivering a significantly lower dose of fibrinolytic drug directly into the thrombus over an extended period of time (12–24 hours) through a multisidehole infusion catheter (**Fig. 1**).[21] The dose administered in prior evaluations of CDT has been approximately one-fourth that given systemically (ie, 20–24 mg of alteplase), although the optimal dosing strategy is being actively investigated. Intrathrombus infusion of tPA theoretically exposes a larger surface area of the clot to thrombolytic drugs.[31] This mechanism has been suggested by Schmitz-Rode and colleagues,[32,33] who showed proximal vortex formation by obstructing emboli preventing a systemically administered drug from making effective contact with the embolus.

An alternative to standard infusion catheters is the EkoSonic Endovascular System infusion catheter (EKOS Corp, Bothell, WA).[27] This drug delivery catheter, cleared by the US Food and Drug Administration (FDA) for use within the PAs, uses microsonic (high-frequency, low-intensity ultrasound) energy delivered through the catheter core. The ultrasound energy is hypothesized to alter the local architecture of the fibrin clot (ie, loosen and separate fibrin to enhance clot permeability while increasing available plasminogen activation receptor sites for tPA) and drive the thrombolytic agent deep into the blood clot to accelerate thrombolysis.[34] ULTIMA and SEATTLE II investigators used ultrasonography-assisted CDT but did not assess whether it was more effective than standard CDT.[26,27] In the PERFECT registry, there was no difference in technical or clinical success between ultrasonography-assisted and standard CDT.[28] A retrospective study by Liang and colleagues,[35] comparing ultrasonography-assisted thrombolysis and standard CDT for the

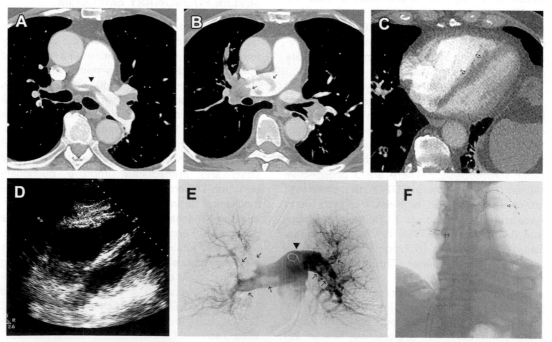

Fig. 1. A 78-year-old man presenting with acute dyspnea. Initial evaluation revealed a dyspneic patient with a heart rate of 90 beats/min, a blood pressure of 140/87 mm Hg, and oxygen saturation of 85% to 90% on room air. (A, B) Axial computed tomography (CT) pulmonary angiography images show acute saddle embolus (*arrowhead*) extending into the left and right main pulmonary arteries and their lobar branches (*arrows*). (C) Axial CT image at the level of the ventricles shows a severely dilated right ventricle and flattening of the interventricular septum (*open arrows*); the right ventricle/left ventricle ratio on 4-chamber reformatted imaging was 2:1. (D) Echocardiography performed at the emergency department shows a severely dilated and hypokinetic right ventricle. The cardiac biomarker levels were increased. The patient was transferred to the interventional radiology suite and pulmonary angiography (E) showed large filling defects in the main (*arrowhead*), left, and right pulmonary arteries and several lobar and segmental branches (*arrows*). (F) CDT was performed by dual-catheter infusion into the left (*open arrow*) and right (*double arrow*) pulmonary arteries using a femoral access and EKOS infusion system.

treatment of acute PE showed no statistical differences in clinical and hemodynamic outcomes or procedural complication rates between these two methods. At present, it is unknown whether ultrasonography-assisted CDT offers improved fibrinolysis and safety compared with standard multisidehole infusion catheters, because there are no randomized trials comparing these two techniques.[22]

CONTRAINDICATIONS FOR CATHETER-DIRECTED INTERVENTION

There are relative and absolute contraindications to catheter-directed therapy in the pulmonary circulation.[36,37] Because coexistent pulmonary hypertension is a relative contraindication to pulmonary angiography and patients referred for interventional treatment of PE are likely to have at least some degree of pulmonary hypertension and RV strain, the degree of pulmonary hypertension and underlying cardiopulmonary disease state should be assessed before performing pulmonary angiography. Several techniques can be used to mitigate risk in such cases and are discussed later. Left bundle branch block on electrocardiogram (ECG) is another relative contraindication for pulmonary angiography and intervention. Induced right bundle branch block in these patients may result in complete heart block. External pacing pads or a transvenous pacing catheter should be readily available in such cases. The risk of contrast reaction in patients with a prior history can be addressed with emergent prophylactic premedication[38]; however, this risk is not prohibitive in most cases because the procedure can be performed without contrast injection.

Because of the risk of major hemorrhage, local CDT may be contraindicated in patients with recent (<10 days) major general surgery, deep organ biopsy or puncture, or obstetric delivery; recent (<10 days) gastrointestinal bleeding; major internal bleeding within the past 6 months; recent major trauma; severe arterial hypertension (systolic blood pressure >200 mm Hg or diastolic blood pressure >110 mm Hg); and hemorrhagic retinopathy. In addition, active bleeding, recent (within 2 months) cerebrovascular accident, recent (within 3 months) intracranial or intraspinal surgery, and presence of other active intracranial processes (aneurysm, vascular malformation, or neoplasm) have been considered by some to be absolute contraindications for thrombolytic drug administration. However, in such cases, individualized risk assessment is essential through a multidisciplinary consensus, taking into account thrombus burden and location, imaging and biomarker results, bleeding risk, and prognosis (Table 1). In the current era, patients with severe PE with these contraindications and no other options have been successfully treated with catheter-directed therapy.[20,28] In patients with recent surgeries, it might be informative to contact the surgeon in an effort to estimate the bleeding risk, because some surgeries might carry a lower than anticipated risk of bleeding.

PROCEDURE PREPARATION

Interventionalists should review available diagnostic imaging studies to determine the relevant vascular anatomy, location/extent of pulmonary emboli, and presence/extent of deep venous

Table 1
Directions for intermediate-risk pulmonary embolism management

Intermediate-Risk PE Type/Presentation	Need for Treatment Escalation with CDT
Intermediate-high-risk PE bordering on high risk: very sick patients with signs of organ hypoperfusion (eg, increased lactate and liver enzyme levels) or severe RV dysfunction	Frequently If there is a saddle embolus, consult cardiothoracic surgery, because embolectomy might be a viable option; systemic lysis may also be an option
Intermediate-high-risk PE (sPESI ≥1, with evidence of both RV dysfunction and increased cardiac biomarker levels)	Possibly; particularly if there are concerning signs such as a severely hypokinetic RV and occlusive central clot, particularly if there is a lack of improvement in symptoms and hemodynamics with anticoagulation alone, and low bleeding risk
Intermediate-low-risk PE (sPESI ≥1, with absence of both or evidence of either RV dysfunction or increased cardiac biomarker levels)	Infrequently May choose to undergo CDT in young or active patients with central thrombus and low risk of bleeding

thrombosis, which could influence approach and choice of access site.[39] If not already performed, limited preprocedural lower extremity ultrasonography is advised. Review of ECG findings provides information on the risk of arrhythmias and heart block.

Before starting the procedure, the operator should ensure the preparedness of the team, availability of all required equipment (**Table 2**),

and the presence of an appropriate support team.[39] Discussing the procedure plan and anticipated course of the procedure and complications with the assistants, technologists, nurses, and anesthesia staff is helpful to ensure the readiness of the interventional team. If anesthesia is required, a specialized cardiac anesthesiologist may be considered given the tenuous state of the RV. Induction, sedation, and excessive

Table 2
Interventional pulmonary embolism treatment tray: equipment needed for catheter-based therapy

Equipment	Purpose
Vascular Access	
Vascular sheath (5–6 F, short)	To secure initial vascular access Will require 2 sheaths if plan for bilateral CDT
Micropuncture needle kit (Boston Scientific, Natick, MA or Cook Medical Inc, Bloomington, IN)	To reduce the risk of access site–related complications
Ultrasonography for guidance and sterile ultrasound probe cover	To reduce the risk of access site–related complications
Pulmonary Catheterization and Angiography	
Cobra, angled pigtail, or straight pigtail catheters (100 cm)	To catheterize the pulmonary artery
Balloon-tipped pulmonary artery catheter	Can be helpful in cases of severe tricuspid regurgitation or a severely dilated right ventricle
Pigtail catheter	To perform pulmonary angiography
Rosen wire (0.035 inch, 260 cm) Wholey wire (0.035 inch, 260 cm)	Start with an exchange-length medium-stiffness wire, to provide stability
Amplatz wire (0.035 inch, 260 cm)	Stiff wire to provide increased stability for catheter exchange or escalation to mechanical thrombectomy
Long flexor sheath (5–6 F, 55 cm)	To provide a stable access for CDT
Medications	
Intravenous unfractionated heparin (300–500 units/h through the sheath)	To maintain subtherapeutic anticoagulation and prevent perisheath clot formation
tPA (alteplase; Genentech, South San Francisco, CA)	To perform thrombolysis; recommended total infusion dose is 1–2 mg/h for a total dose of 24 mg (half the dose through each catheter for bilateral catheters)
Contrast agent (nonionic, low-osmolality contrast)	To perform angiography
Infusion Catheters	
Cragg-McNamara Valved Infusion Catheter (Covidien, Plymouth, MN)	Multisidehole catheter for intraclot infusion of thrombolytic agent
UniFuse Infusion Catheter (Angiodynamics, Latham, NY)	Multisidehole catheter for intraclot infusion of thrombolytic agent
Ultrasonography-assisted EkoSonic Endovascular System (EKOS, Bothell, WA)	Multisidehole catheter with an ultrasound-emitting wire to perform ultrasonography-assisted CDT
Other Devices	
External pacemaker, internal venous pacemaker	To treat complete heart block if this complication occurs

positive pressure ventilation can reduce preload and precipitate hemodynamic collapse.

In patients with high-risk PE and patients with intermediate-risk PE at high risk for deterioration, the team should be ready to initiate lifesaving maneuvers such as mechanical circulatory support and/or rescue embolectomy, which may require a hybrid operating room.

PROCEDURE

A variety of methods can be used to catheterize the PA depending on the operator's experience and preference. Ultrasonography-guided frontwall femoral or jugular puncture is preferred in most patients who are candidates for CDT or thrombectomy. If dual catheter infusions are required, a second femoral or jugular vein access (in the same vein) is acceptable. The right internal jugular approach may be preferred in the presence of a large thrombus in the inferior vena cava (IVC), iliac vein, and/or femoral vein. Antecubital veins (basilic, cephalic, brachial) can be used as well when other access sites are limited. After obtaining venous access, a 5-F or 6-F angled or straight pigtail or cobra-shaped catheter is advanced over a guidewire in a stepwise fashion through the right atrium (RA) and into the RV and main PA. If large-bore devices are planned, then a balloon-tipped catheter that is floated into the PA may avoid catching an RV chordae that subsequently could be damaged by large-sheath passage. The balloon-tipped catheters can also be helpful when other catheters cannot access the RV outflow tract because of severe tricuspid regurgitation or a severely dilated right ventricle. The ECG should be continuously monitored to detect induced cardiac arrhythmias.

Measurement of RA pressures (RAPs) and RV end-diastolic pressures, as well as systolic and mean PAPs, helps determine the risk of angiography and obtain baseline preintervention pressure readings. In addition, pulmonary arterial oxygen saturation can be sampled to measure cardiac output via the Fick principle. When the systolic PAP exceeds 55 mm Hg, or the RAP/RV EDP is greater than 20 mm Hg, the risk associated with pulmonary angiography is increased. Lower injection rates and the use of nonionic contrast media can mitigate the risk.[36] In such circumstances, an injection rate of 10 to 15 mL/s can be considered. If the preintervention computed tomography is adequate, angiography can be deferred altogether.

After pressure measurement and angiography, the guidewire can be exchanged for a stiff wire (eg, 0.035-inch Rosen or Amplatz) to provide stability for subsequent long vascular sheath placement. This sheath allows secure access of the thrombectomy catheter/device to the PA and stability of infusion catheters during thrombolysis. Multisidehole catheters (infusion lengths of 10–20 cm) are passed over the wires via the sheaths and embedded within the thrombus. The tip is most commonly placed in the interlobar artery. The recommended total tPA infusion rate is 1 to 2 mg/h, for a total dose of 24 mg. Some operators advocate boluses of tPA of 1 to 4 mg during initial catheter placement. A common protocol infuses alteplase at a rate of 0.5 to 1 mg/h through each PA catheter if bilateral catheters are used.[27]

Following catheter placement, the vascular sheaths and infusion catheters should be secured in place with sutures and dressing. Patients should be transferred to monitored beds. The postprocedural order set should include detailed instructions for the observation period and specific criteria for nursing staff to alert the physicians (Table 3).[40] PAP measurements can be obtained through the sheath during the monitoring period if a long sheath is used. Fibrinogen levels can be monitored during the infusion but do not clearly correlate with bleeding and outcomes.[41] However, when fibrinogen levels decrease to less than 100 to 150 mg/dL, the operator may choose to reduce/discontinue the infusion, and/or transfuse with fresh frozen plasma or cryoprecipitate. The thrombolytic infusion should be stopped if the patient has a clinically significant bleed. Other criteria for discontinuation of thrombolytic infusion include (1) reduction in PAP with subjective and objective clinical improvement (eg, diminished dyspnea, heart rate reduction, improved systemic blood pressure, improved oxygen saturation); (2) posttreatment angiography showing improved pulmonary blood flow; (3) echocardiography showing improved RV function.

During the procedure, full anticoagulation may be continued. However, once the thrombolytic infusion has been initiated, a subtherapeutic heparin dose (eg, 300–500 units/h through the vascular sheath, with a goal partial thromboplastin time <2 times the institutional normal), reduces perisheath clot formation and minimizes bleeding.

There are no data to support the routine placement of IVC filters for patients with intermediate-risk PE who can be anticoagulated.[42] Patients with high-risk PE should receive IVC filters regardless of anticoagulation status, based on lower mortality associations with IVC filters in the International Cooperative Pulmonary Embolism Registry (ICOPER) and a national inpatient database survey.[43,44]

Table 3
Postprocedural infusion instructions

Instructions	Rationale
Keep patient on complete bed rest with legs extended (femoral access)	Minimize the risk of access site complications and dislodging the catheter
Keep patient fasting (or on clear liquid diet)	Depending on clinical status, other comorbidities, risk of aspiration, expected risk of bleeding and need to an emergency surgery, intubation, or reintervention to prevent or decrease the risk of aspiration
Check vascular access sites for signs of bleeding and hematoma formation	Early detection of access site complications
Perform serial neurologic tests (every 2–4 h)	Early detection of intracranial bleeding complications
Monitor complete blood count, fibrinogen, partial thromboplastin time (eg, every 4 h)	Early detection of complications (bleeding, acute anemia, supratherapeutic levels of anticoagulation, hypofibrinogenemia)
Remove sheaths and perform manual compression for hemostasis (30–45 min) after thrombolytic infusion is stopped	This is the correct/recommended period to allow for rapidly obtaining hemostasis while minimizing the total amount of time that the patient is not therapeutically anticoagulated

FOLLOW-UP CARE

Once CDT is completed, full therapeutic anticoagulation should be resumed, unless contraindicated. Details of sheath removal are given in **Table 3**. Interventionalists should participate in longitudinal follow-up. Outpatient follow-up ensures adequate anticoagulation and recognition of signs and symptoms of long-term complications such as unresolved dyspnea and exercise intolerance. If a temporary IVC filter was inserted during the procedure, the patient should be scheduled for filter retrieval once filtration is no longer indicated to spare patients the potential risks associated with long-term filter implantation.

SUMMARY

Catheter-directed therapy is gaining traction in the medical community as a treatment option for patients with high-risk and intermediate-risk PE; however, the practice cannot be routinely recommended based on current data. Robust randomized trials with clinically relevant short-term and long-term outcomes are needed to assess the clinical utility of CDT in patients with intermediate-risk PE.

REFERENCES

1. Tapson VF. Acute pulmonary embolism. N Engl J Med 2008;358(10):1037–52.
2. Pulido T, Aranda A, Zevallos MA, et al. Pulmonary embolism as a cause of death in patients with heart disease: an autopsy study. Chest 2006;129(5):1282–7.
3. Park B, Messina L, Dargon P, et al. Recent trends in clinical outcomes and resource utilization for pulmonary embolism in the United States: findings from the nationwide inpatient sample. Chest 2009;136(4):983–90.
4. Horlander KT, Mannino DM, Leeper KV. Pulmonary embolism mortality in the United States, 1979-1998: an analysis using multiple-cause mortality data. Arch Intern Med 2003;163(14):1711–7.
5. Konstantinides S, Torbicki A, Agnelli G, et al. 2014 ESC guidelines on the diagnosis and management of acute pulmonary embolism. Eur Heart J 2014; 35(43):3033–69, 3069a–3069k.
6. Sista AK, Miller LE, Kahn SR, et al. Persistent right ventricular dysfunction, functional capacity limitation, exercise intolerance, and quality of life impairment following pulmonary embolism: systematic review with meta-analysis. Vasc Med 2016;1:7.
7. Klok FA, van Kralingen KW, van Dijk AP, et al. Quality of life in long-term survivors of acute pulmonary embolism. Chest 2010;138(6):1432–40.
8. Fanikos J, Piazza G, Zayaruzny M, et al. Long-term complications of medical patients with hospital-acquired venous thromboembolism. Thromb Haemost 2009;102(4):688–93.
9. Piazza G, Goldhaber SZ. Chronic thromboembolic pulmonary hypertension. N Engl J Med 2011; 364(4):351–60.
10. Casazza F, Becattini C, Bongarzoni A, et al. Clinical features and short term outcomes of patients with acute pulmonary embolism. The Italian Pulmonary Embolism Registry (IPER). Thromb Res 2012; 130(6):847–52.

11. Jaff MR, McMurtry MS, Archer SL, et al. Management of massive and submassive pulmonary embolism, iliofemoral deep vein thrombosis, and chronic thromboembolic pulmonary hypertension: a scientific statement from the American Heart Association. Circulation 2011;123(16): 1788–830.

12. Wood KE. Major pulmonary embolism: review of a pathophysiologic approach to the golden hour of hemodynamically significant pulmonary embolism. Chest 2002;121(3):877–905.

13. Kabrhel C, Jaff MR, Channick RN, et al. A multidisciplinary pulmonary embolism response team. Chest 2013;144(5):1738–9.

14. Sista A, Friedman OA, Horowitz JM, et al. Building a pulmonary embolism lysis practice. Endovasc Today 2013;12:61–4.

15. Kearon C, Akl EA, Comerota AJ, et al. Antithrombotic therapy for VTE disease: antithrombotic therapy and prevention of thrombosis: American College of Chest Physicians evidence-based clinical practice guidelines. Chest 2012;141(2_suppl): e419S–494.

16. Kearon C, Akl EA, Ornelas J, et al. Antithrombotic therapy for VTE disease: CHEST guideline and expert panel report. Chest 2016;149(2):315–52.

17. Goldhaber SZ. Surgical pulmonary embolectomy: the resurrection of an almost discarded operation. Tex Heart Inst J 2013;40(1):5.

18. Neely RC, Byrne JG, Gosev I, et al. Surgical embolectomy for acute massive and submassive pulmonary embolism in a series of 115 patients. Ann Thorac Surg 2015;100(4):1245–52.

19. Worku B, Gulkarov I, Girardi LN, et al. Pulmonary embolectomy In the treatment of submassive and massive pulmonary embolism. Cardiology 2014; 129(2):106–10.

20. Kuo WT, Gould MK, Louie JD, et al. Catheter-directed therapy for the treatment of massive pulmonary embolism: systematic review and meta-analysis of modern techniques. J Vasc Interv Radiol 2009;20(11):1431–40.

21. Kuo WT. Endovascular therapy for acute pulmonary embolism. J Vasc Interv Radiol 2012;23(2):167–79.e4.

22. Sista AK, Horowitz JM, Goldhaber SZ. Four key questions surrounding thrombolytic therapy for submassive pulmonary embolism. Vasc Med 2016; 21(1):47–52.

23. Chatterjee S, Chakraborty A, Weinberg I, et al. Thrombolysis for pulmonary embolism and risk of all-cause mortality, major bleeding, and intracranial hemorrhage: a meta-analysis. JAMA 2014;311(23): 2414–21.

24. Marti C, John G, Konstantinides S, et al. Systemic thrombolytic therapy for acute pulmonary embolism: a systematic review and meta-analysis. Eur Heart J 2015;36(10):605–14.

25. Meyer G, Vicaut E, Danays T, et al. Fibrinolysis for patients with intermediate-risk pulmonary embolism. N Engl J Med 2014;370(15):1402–11.

26. Kucher N, Boekstegers P, Muller OJ, et al. Randomized, controlled trial of ultrasound-assisted catheter-directed thrombolysis for acute intermediate-risk pulmonary embolism. Circulation 2014;129(4):479–86.

27. Piazza G, Hohlfelder B, Jaff MR, et al. A prospective, single-arm, multicenter trial of ultrasound-facilitated, catheter-directed, low-dose fibrinolysis for acute massive and submassive pulmonary embolism: the SEATTLE II Study. JACC Cardiovasc Interv 2015;8(10):1382–92.

28. Kuo WT, Banerjee A, Kim PS, et al. Pulmonary Embolism Response to Fragmentation, Embolectomy, and Catheter Thrombolysis (PERFECT): initial results from a prospective multicenter registry. Chest 2015;148(3):667–73.

29. Goldhaber SZ, Come P, Lee R, et al. Alteplase versus heparin in acute pulmonary embolism: randomised trial assessing right-ventricular function and pulmonary perfusion. Lancet 1993;341(8844): 507–11.

30. Nakazawa K, Tajima H, Murata S, et al. Catheter fragmentation of acute massive pulmonary thromboembolism: distal embolisation and pulmonary arterial pressure elevation. Br J Radiol 2014;81: 848–54.

31. Uflacker R. Interventional therapy for pulmonary embolism. J Vasc Interv Radiol 2001;12(2):147–64.

32. Verstraete M, Miller G, Bounameaux H, et al. Intravenous and intrapulmonary recombinant tissue-type plasminogen activator in the treatment of acute massive pulmonary embolism. Circulation 1988;77(2):353–60.

33. Schmitz-Rode T, Kilbinger M, Günther RW. Simulated flow pattern in massive pulmonary embolism: significance for selective intrapulmonary thrombolysis. Cardiovasc Interv Radiol 1998;21(3): 199–204.

34. Chamsuddin A, Nazzal L, Kang B, et al. Catheter-directed thrombolysis with the Endowave system in the treatment of acute massive pulmonary embolism: a retrospective multicenter case series. J Vasc Interv Radiol 2008;19(3):372–6.

35. Liang NL, Avgerinos ED, Marone LK, et al. Comparative outcomes of ultrasound-assisted thrombolysis and standard catheter-directed thrombolysis in the treatment of acute pulmonary embolism. Vasc endovascular Surg 2016;50(6):405–10.

36. Mauro MA, Murphy KPJ, Thomson KR, et al. Image-guided interventions. Philadelphia: Saunders Elsevier; 2014.

37. Farquharson S. Pulmonary artery thrombectomy and thrombolysis. In: Taslakian B, Al-Kutoubi A, Hoballah JJ, editors. Procedural dictations in

image-guided intervention. Switzerland: Springer International Publishing; 2016. p. 545–51.

38. Taslakian B, Sebaaly MG, Al-Kutoubi A. Patient evaluation and preparation in vascular and interventional radiology: what every interventional radiologist should know (part 2: patient preparation and medications). Cardiovasc Interv Radiol 2016; 39(4):489–99.

39. Taslakian B, Sebaaly MG, Al-Kutoubi A. Patient evaluation and preparation in vascular and interventional radiology: what every interventional radiologist should know (part 1: patient assessment and laboratory tests). Cardiovasc Interv Radiol 2016;39(3):325–33.

40. Taslakian B, Sridhar D. Post-procedural care in interventional radiology: what every interventional radiologist should know—part I: standard post-procedural instructions and follow-up care. Cardiovasc Interv Radiol 2017;40:481–95.

41. Poorthuis MH, Brand EC, Hazenberg CE, et al. Plasma fibrinogen level as a potential predictor of hemorrhagic complications after catheter-directed thrombolysis for peripheral arterial occlusions. J Vasc Surg 2017;65:1519–27.e26.

42. Mismetti P, Laporte S, Pellerin O, et al. Effect of a retrievable inferior vena cava filter plus anticoagulation vs anticoagulation alone on risk of recurrent pulmonary embolism: a randomized clinical trial. JAMA 2015;313(16):1627–35.

43. Kucher N, Rossi E, De Rosa M, et al. Massive pulmonary embolism. Circulation 2006;113(4):577–82.

44. Stein PD, Matta F, Keyes DC, et al. Impact of vena cava filters on in-hospital case fatality rate from pulmonary embolism. Am J Med 2012;125(5):478–84.

Catheter-Based Embolectomy for Acute Pulmonary Embolism

Devices, Technical Considerations, Risks, and Benefits

Wissam A. Jaber, MD*, Michael C. McDaniel, MD

KEYWORDS

- Pulmonary embolism • Pulmonary embolectomy • Catheter therapy • Catheter-directed therapy
- Percutaneous intervention

KEY POINTS

- Percutaneous pulmonary embolectomy can be useful in high-risk patients with contraindication to thrombolytics, although data are limited.
- Understanding the anatomy and defining the location of pulmonary thrombi are key to a successful procedure.
- Given that all techniques are challenging and achieve at best a partial thrombus removal, more comparative outcomes and technological research are needed.

INTRODUCTION

The cornerstone for treatment of pulmonary embolism (PE) is anticoagulation. Other treatment modalities, like surgery, catheter therapy, or thrombolysis, remain controversial, especially in the absence of cardiogenic shock. With the recent rise in the use of catheter-based treatments for PE patients, interventionalists should become familiar with all available options and techniques.

This text reviews the general indications and principles of nonlytic catheter treatment of PE, reviews the available data, describes the general techniques of catheter placement in the pulmonary artery (PA) branches, and then describes specific catheters used in PE treatment.

INDICATIONS

Patients who are hemodynamically compromised (high-risk or massive PE) have a high mortality rate with anticoagulation alone and may benefit from a more advanced treatment modality. Although systemic thrombolysis is usually indicated for these patients, at least a third have some contraindication to systemic thrombolytics.[1] Moreover, up to 10% of patients who receive systemic thrombolysis remain in shock.[2] For these patients, surgical embolectomy should be considered. Surgical expertise is often limited, however, to selected centers and there can be high morbidity and mortality, especially in patients who have failed thrombolytics. As such, percutaneous pulmonary embolectomy is

---

Conflict of Interest: W.A. Jaber has received an unrestricted research grant from Inari Medical; Dr M.C. McDaniel has no conflicts of interest.

Division of Cardiology, Emory University School of Medicine, 550 Peachtree Street, MOT 6th Floor, Atlanta, GA 30308, USA

* Corresponding author.

E-mail address: Wissam.jaber@emory.edu

recommended for many high-risk PE patients with contraindications to thrombolysis and/or failure of thrombolysis if the expertise is available at the treatment facility (class IIa, level of evidence [LOE] C).[3,4]

A more controversial indication for catheter-based embolectomy is the presence of right heart strain without shock (intermediate-risk or submassive PE). A majority of these patients should continue to be treated with anticoagulation alone, and more advanced therapy (thrombolysis, catheter-based therapy, or surgery) should be reserved for those at the upper end of the risk spectrum and at low risk for complications from such therapies (class IIb, LOE C).[3,4] Patients with significant symptoms and persistent desaturation despite anticoagulation for a few days may also potentially benefit from invasive therapy that targets occlusive thrombi in main PA branches, although the proof for such benefit is currently anecdotal.[5]

In the appropriate clinical scenario, anatomic criteria must also be met when considering catheter therapy. Totally or subtotally occluded central, lobar, or interlobar branches should be the targets of therapy, rather than segmental branches.

For patients without a contraindication to thrombolysis, systemic or catheter-directed thrombolysis should be considered before catheter embolectomy given the higher LOE for the former compared with the latter.[6] In the presence of hemodynamic compromise or if a patient is at risk for worsening clinical status and in the presence of contraindication to thrombolysis, catheter-based embolectomy can be an attractive option, especially as an alternative to surgical embolectomy.

Given the lack of data and the absence of a standard approach to catheter embolectomy, selection of patients for such treatment is best undertaken after multidisciplinary discussions among specialists with expertise in PE treatment and in centers familiar with its techniques.[7]

CHALLENGES

All percutaneous PE treatment modalities face the following common challenges:

- Attempting to remove large, frequently organized thrombi with devices limited in size
- Difficult manipulation through large spaces that are often tortuous
- Thrombi frequently involving many branches that are difficult to visualize and navigate

- Risk of vascular complication both at the access site and the pulmonary bed in an anticoagulated patient
- Unclear endpoints to determine the completion of the procedure (PA pressure, right ventricular size, thrombus reduction, PA blood flow, clinical status, and so forth)
- Lack of scientific evidence: data behind percutaneous PE thrombectomy are limited to case reports or retrospective case series. As illustrated in a metanalysis by Kuo and colleagues[8] of available catheter-based PE treatment studies, clinical success was achieved in 86%, but there was significant heterogeneity in the definition of success, and most of the thrombectomy cases also included some form of catheter-directed thrombolytic therapy.
- No currently available device is able to remove the majority of the PE. The goal of treatment is usually to remove or macerate as much thrombi as possible to allow better pulmonary perfusion and hence hemodynamic stabilization or symptomatic improvement.
- None of the devices currently on the market is approved or cleared by the US Food and Drug Administration (FDA) for PE treatment.

TECHNICAL CONSIDERATIONS
Venous Access

Managing access is a prerequisite for a successful thrombectomy. Most complications of catheter treatment of PE are related to access site (injury or hematoma), especially when there is concomitant thrombolytic use, which is commonly performed in conjunction with catheter thrombectomy.[8] Access should be obtained under direct ultrasonographic guidance, which is also helpful in ruling out venous thrombi at the access site. Either jugular or femoral veins may be accessed for pulmonary thrombectomy, with differing advantages and disadvantages depending on the individual device used.

In femoral venous access, venous angiography is performed to ensure adequate venous size and absence of thrombi. In cases of the iliac vein appearing focally small/compressed (as in May-Thurner syndrome), it can still be frequently crossed by a large sheath safely, but care should be exerted not to push against resistance, and sheath advancement should be directly observed under fluoroscopy. General advantages of femoral access with large bore thrombectomy devices include comfort for the operator in working from this position, an easily compressible access site, and good ability to direct wires into either lung. Some technical details of placement of large bore devices from a right internal jugular approach are reviewed later.

After completion of the case, hemostasis can be successfully achieved in the majority of cases using manual compression, even in the presence of full anticoagulation. In large bore access, a figure-of-8 suture can be sufficient for hemostasis,[9] although deployment of a suture-mediated closure device (preclosure) prior to entry point dilatation has been successfully used with few reported complications.[10] In the authors' practice, when using preclosure for large bore venous access, use of just a single 6 French (F) Perclose (Abbott Vascular, Santa Clara, California) is favored, regardless of sheath size with subsequent manual compression for 5 minutes to 15 minutes. This differs from the authors' practice in arterial preclosure, where 2 devices for sheath sizes of 14F or above are often used.

Right Heart Catheterization

Performing a right heart catheterization at the beginning of the procedure with documentation of baseline right atrial pressure, PA pressure, and PA saturation (as a surrogate for cardiac output) is important for evaluation of the hemodynamic impact of the acute PE, to assess the risk of the procedure, and to be able to assess the effect of the treatment on the final hemodynamics. Importantly, when hemodynamics assessed with right heart catheterization are not very deranged and the patient does not have hypoxic respiratory failure, strong consideration should be given to aborting the embolectomy procedure.

Anticoagulation During the Procedure

Although the protocol varies between different centers, anticoagulation during the procedure is always recommended. The authors usually continue anticoagulation with systemic heparin (or argatroban in patient with heparin-induced thrombocytopenia) except for patients who had just received systemic doses of thrombolytics. It may be helpful to keep the activated clotting time above 200 seconds by giving additional anticoagulant doses as needed. Reversing or stopping anticoagulation for sheath removal is rarely necessary to obtain hemostasis.

Pulmonary Angiogram

Studying the CT pulmonary angiogram is important in preparing for the invasive procedure. Information obtained includes the location of the thrombi, involved branches, potential targets for treatment, choice of thrombectomy device, and best projection during angiography to help maximize a PA branching angle for catheter navigation.

It is common to start the procedure with a 6F or 7F venous sheath, perform venous angiography, and then proceed with right heart catheterization using a 6F angled pigtail catheter or a 7F balloon-tipped catheter. Use of the balloon-tipped catheter to cross from the right atrium to the PA is important when there is a plan to use stiff wires for catheter exchanges or when using large sheath advancements into the PA, given that the balloon-tipped catheter is less likely than nonballoon catheters to become entrapped underneath a tricuspid valve papillary muscle or cord, thus avoiding damage to the tricuspid apparatus.

Once the catheter is in the PA and after pressure measurement, a selective right and left PA angiogram is performed. A main PA angiogram requires a higher amount of contrast injection and is usually not necessary especially when a CT angiogram had been performed. A pigtail or a multipurpose catheter with a J-tipped or Wholey guide wire may be needed to select the right PA. In patients with significant right ventricular dysfunction and reduced cardiac output, manual injection of contrast is all that is needed for adequate visualization. In less sick patients with normal cardiac output, using a power injector may be necessary for adequate opacification of the PA, with volume up to 30 mL of contrast injected in the right and left main PA at a rate rise of 15 mL/s. In patients with severe pulmonary hypertension, where power injection may precipitate worsening right ventricular failure and in whom manual injection in the main PA branches does not yield adequate visualization, selective manual injections in lobar/interlobar branches may be helpful. Fig. 1 shows an example of bilateral PA angiograms performed with power injection and digital subtraction.

In patients who are able to hold their breath for a few seconds, digital subtraction may be helpful for better opacification and less contrast dose injection. Otherwise regular angiography is performed. If available, biplane angiography is preferred over single plane. When not available, the right PA angiogram is initially performed in an anteroposterior or slight right anterior oblique projection, and the left PA angiogram in a

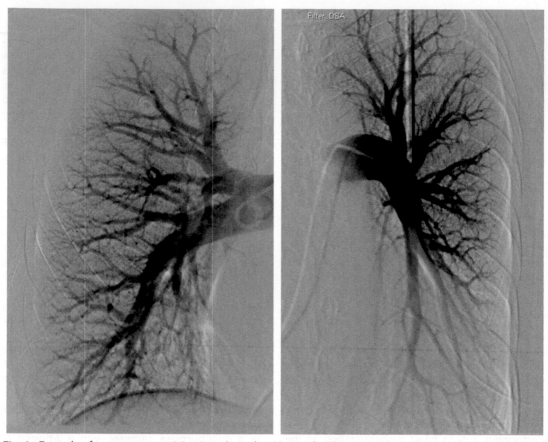

Fig. 1. Example of separate power injections through a 6F pigtail catheter into the right and left PA (*left* and *right panel*, respectively), done with digital subtraction. Notice the absence of filling defects and the presence of uniform perfusion in the peripheral segments.

10° to 20° of left anterior oblique projection. When a single projection is used, a repeat angiogram in a different angle is sometimes needed to help separate the distal branches. The contralateral oblique projection is valuable for separating out branches of the lower lobes.

In interpreting the pulmonary angiogram, it is important to not only focus on the location and size of the filling defects representing PA thrombi but also to note the perfusion of the respective lung segments and lobes (**Fig. 2**) by continuing cineangiography into the early venous phase.

Pulmonary Arterial Branch to Treat: Selection and Technique

The best PA branch to treat is the one that is most obstructed, identified angiographically by large occlusive thrombus burden and by a lack of peripheral perfusion to the corresponding lung segments. The branch has to also be technically accessible. The main PA or interlobar branches are the most common targets (see **Fig. 2**; **Fig. 3**).

After the angiogram is performed and a decision is made to proceed with thrombectomy, the access sheath is exchanged over a long 0.035-in wire to the appropriate sheath size based on the catheter intended to be used (different catheter options discussed later) If the PA has already been accessed using a balloon-tipped catheter, the sheath can be exchanged with a long wire in the PA to avoid recrossing the right ventricle.

Regardless of what device or technique is used to perform the thrombectomy, selective engagement and safe wiring of the target branch is a prerequisite, starting with adequate visualization through angiography. Over a non-traumatic J-tipped wire, a steerable catheter (for example multipurpose or Judkins right 4) is advanced to the thrombus. Further advancement beyond the thrombus requires selective low-volume contrast injection through the

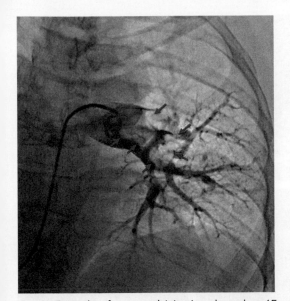

Fig. 2. Example of a manual injection through a 6F pigtail catheter in the left main PA showing significant thrombi (filling defects [*red arrows*]). The reduced flow in the left lung in this patient with large PE allowed for adequate opacification with less than 10 mL of manual contrast injection. Note the absent perfusion in the left upper lobe.

catheter tip to document both adequate placement and size of the selected branch. The branch has to be big enough to allow a J-tipped wire for catheter exchanges and to allow the appropriate thrombectomy catheter to be delivered (see **Fig. 3**). In tortuous vessels, a nontraumatic tip 0.018 wire may be gently advanced and steered by a small profile catheter (eg, Angled Glidecath [Terumo, Somerset, New Jersey]). Given their tendency to cause distal perforation, straight or angled hydrophilic wires (eg, Glidewire [Terumo]) should be used with utmost caution and only when anatomy is very well understood, preferably in large vessels. Less-traumatic Wholey wires may be somewhat safer, although the lack of a J-tip still can predispose to guidance of devices into small branches. Once satisfied with the distal position of the catheter, the operator can then exchange the diagnostic catheter to the desired treatment catheter over an exchange length wire. The authors have found that the Safe-T-J Rosen 0.035-in exchange guide wire (Cook Medical, Bloomington, Indiana) offers enough support for large catheter exchange while having a safe short floppy tip with a small 1.5-mm radius, suitable for placement in subsegmental PA branches.

SPECIFIC CATHETERS AND TECHNIQUES

The currently used and described catheters and techniques in the treatment of PE are discussed. Older devices that are no longer in use are not discussed.

Maceration with Pigtail Rotation Catheter and Ballooning

As described in a series of 20 patients with massive PE,[11] clot maceration can be performed using a modified pigtail catheter where the guide wire exits from a side hole at the outer curvature of the pigtail loop, leaving the loop free to rotate around the wire. The rotation is performed manually, with the hope of breaking down the fresh thrombus into small fragments that can then embolize downstream where the cross-sectional area of smaller arterial branches is larger than the proximal PA, allowing for some improvement in the forward blood flow. Peripheral balloons can also be used for the same purpose, with care to make sure the balloons are smaller than the arterial diameter (usually <16-mm balloons.) These techniques may be helpful in hypotensive patients with totally occluded proximal PA branch, where maceration can establish some forward flow and partially decompress the right ventricle until further treatment, for example, local thrombolysis, takes effect. They run the risk, however, of worsening obstruction by squeezing or embolizing thrombi into previously patent branches. It is not clear whether maceration is helpful by itself, because a majority of the reported cases have been performed in conjunction with thrombolytic injection.[11]

Manual Aspiration Through Large Sheath or Catheter

Manual aspiration of part of the thrombus may be attempted through a large (>8F) sheath or a straight guide catheter advanced over the wire directly into the clot or using specialized catheters (eg, Pronto XL 14F Extraction Catheter [Vascular Solutions, Minneapolis, Minnesota]). It is rare to be able to aspirate a significant amount of thrombus just with simple aspiration, because clots are frequently partially organized and hard to squeeze into a small catheter. Inability to aspirate blood through a syringe attached to the exit port of the sheath or catheter may mean that thrombus is stuck at or near the tip of the catheter. Removal of the whole catheter while maintaining negative suction may pull some thrombi. This method often does little to large proximal thrombi but may be helpful in smaller lobar or

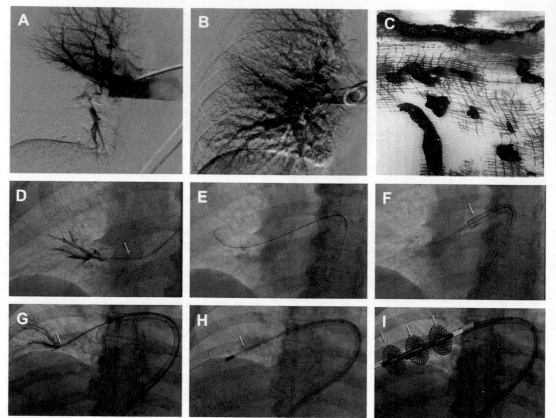

Fig. 3. A case of a patient with submassive PE with acute pulmonary hypertension, treated with the Inari FlowTriever thrombectomy device. (*A*) Baseline pulmonary angiogram shows thrombus obstructing flow to the right middle and lower lobes. (*B*) After treatment, pulmonary angiogram shows restoration of flow. (*C*) Image of thrombus fragments removed. The second and third rows detail the technique of the procedure. (*D*) After baseline pulmonary angiography identifies the target for treatment, the sheath is upsized to 22F and the right PA is accessed again using a balloon-tipped catheter and then exchanged to a multipurpose catheter (*yellow arrow*). The latter is used to cross the thrombus. Gentle injection of contrast through the tip (*red arrow*) documents the location beyond the thrombus and in an artery large enough for advancement of the (*E*) exchange-length wire. (*F*) The 20F aspiration catheter (*arrow*) is then advanced over a dilator to just before the thrombus. (*G*) A multipurpose catheter is then readvanced distally over the wire and injection of contrast is performed (*arrow*) to ensure adequate anatomy for the advancement of the (*H*) FlowTriever catheter (*arrow*). (*I*) The disks are then unsheathed to engage the thrombus (cartoon [*arrows*]). The catheter is retrieved with simultaneous manual aspiration.

segmental branches with total occlusion, especially when due to in-procedure embolization from a treated proximal thrombus.

Rheolytic Thrombectomy

Rheolytic thrombectomy with the Angiojet catheter (Possis, Minneapolis, Minnesota) has been used by some operators for the treatment of massive PE with variable success.[12,13] Technically, its use in the PA is similar to that in the deep veins. While the 8F catheter is advanced slowly into the thrombus over the 0.035-in wire, high-speed saline jets travel backward from the tip of the catheter creating vacuum and thrombus fragmentation effects. While imbedded in the thrombus, the catheter can also be used for pulse delivery of a thrombolytic agent.

In a meta-analysis of published series on invasive treatment of massive PE, Kuo and colleagues[8] found rheolytic thrombectomy associated with a higher incidence of bradycardia, hemolysis, and procedure-related deaths compared with other invasive modalities. The FDA has issued a black-box warning regarding its use in PE treatment.

Aspirex Catheter

The Aspirex catheter (Straub Medical AG, Wangs, Switzerland) is a 6F to 10F over-the-wire fresh thrombus aspiration system. It has been tested in animals for the treatment of acute PE[14] but is not available in the United States. Its mechanism of action consists of a rotating screw inside a catheter with a side window that helps both fragment and aspirate thrombi. There is currently limited experience with this catheter for the treatment of PE.

FlowTriever

The FlowTriever system (Inari Medical, Irvine, California) is a promising technology in large thrombus removal, owing to its large catheter size and engaging disks[5] (see **Fig. 3** for an example of a PE treated with this device). It requires a 22F femoral venous sheath. Once the exchange length wire (like the Rosen wire, described previously) is in the desired PA segmental branch, the 20F aspiration guide catheter is advanced with a dilator through the right heart, up the right or left main PA branches, to just before the thrombus. Care should be exerted while crossing the right heart, and a slight tug/pull of the wire may be needed to negotiate turns. The dilator is then removed and catheter flushed. If the wire has moved from its distal position, a diagnostic 4F or 5F catheter can be reinserted to renegotiate the way past the thrombus and a distal tip injection through the diagnostic catheter performed to ensure appropriate distal location before reinserting the exchange-length wire. The flow

restoration catheter is then advanced inside the 20F aspiration catheter and over the wire across the thrombus. This catheter has 3 nitinol self-expanding disks at the tip that are unsheathed to engage the thrombus once inside the desired PA branch. Simultaneous manual aspiration and withdrawal of the disks through the 20F guide catheter allow for partial thrombus removal. Given the need for continuous aspiration through the large bore device, careful attention should be paid to blood loss during this procedure. Although no data are currently available on this device, an ongoing prospective single arm study is evaluating its safety and effect on right ventricular size in patients with intermediate-risk PE.

Penumbra Indigo

The Indigo embolectomy system (Penumbra, Alameda, California) works on the principle of thrombus aspiration and consists of an 8F angled or straight catheter connected to a suction pump (**Fig. 4**). During aspiration, a separator wire is moved back and forth at the tip to clear the clot and improve the aspiration of the thrombus into the suction canister. The Indigo catheter is cleared for the removal of thrombus

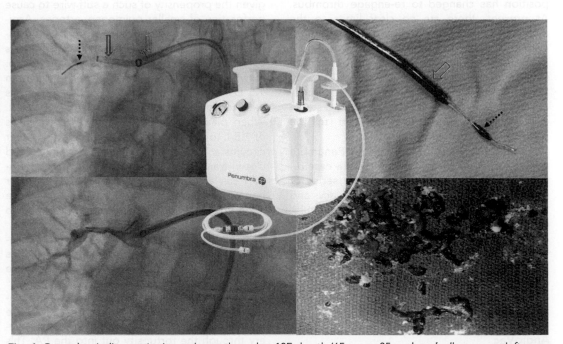

Fig. 4. Penumbra Indigo aspiration catheter: through a 10F sheath (65 cm or 85 cm long [*yellow arrow, left upper panel*]), the 8F guiding catheter (*red block arrows, left and right upper panels*) is advanced into the thrombus (seen on contrast injection of the right middle lobar branch in the left lower panel). Continuous suction is then exerted through an external pump with blood collected in a canister (*inset*), while the separator (*dashed black arrows, left and right upper panels*) is manually advanced and retracted to help break up and move clots in the catheter. The right lower panel shows thrombus fragments collected in the canister. (*Courtesy of* Penumbra Inc, Alameda, CA; with permission).

in the peripheral arterial and venous systems, although it does not carry specific labeling for the pulmonary circulation.

The major benefit of the Indigo system is the small size and ease of delivery into the PA. The Indigo catheter can be placed through a long 65-cm to 90-cm 8F sheath; however, 10F sheaths may be preferred so that angiography can be performed though the sheath with the catheter in place to visualize areas to target for thrombectomy. A regular 0.035-in J-tipped wire or Rosen wire is usually sufficient to advance the sheath into the PA. Despite the small size, the Indigo is capable of large thrombus removal in some circumstances (see **Fig. 4**).

A major drawback to the Indigo catheter system is that it requires aspiration, which can result in large amounts of blood loss without careful technique. To minimize blood loss, the catheter is usually placed more distally into the clot and aspiration performed though a slow pullback while always visualizing the rate of blood aspiration into the canister. There should be little to no blood flow in the canister when the catheter is engaged in the thrombus. Once brisk blood flow returns, this usually means the catheter is no longer engaging the thrombus and the aspiration should be discontinued until the catheter position has changed to re-engage thrombus. At present, there are no clear limits to the amount of blood that can be safely aspirated during a pulmonary embolectomy procedure and must be individualized based on the clinical status of the patient. Cell saver technology can be used to minimize blood loss from the procedure as the aspirated blood is collected in a sterile canister, spun down, and returned to the patient.

The data to support the use of the Penumbra catheter in acute PE are limited to a few case reports.[15] There are no reported case series or randomized trials to detail the efficacy and safety of this device, but a prospective multicenter trial to investigate the safety and efficacy of this catheter in intermediate-risk PE has been developed with plans to start enrollment in late 2017. In addition, the safety, efficacy, and value of Penumbra embolectomy in combination with cell saver technology are unknown and require further study.

AngioVac

The AngioVac catheter (AngioDynamics, Latham, New York) is a large 22F catheter that can remove thrombus through a centrifugal pump and venous reinfusion cannula used in cardiopulmonary bypass (**Fig. 5**). It is cleared by the FDA for the removal of undesirable intravascular material and contains a balloon-expandable funnel-shaped distal tip and an 18F reinfusion cannula. This creates a venous bypass circuit with a large filter in between to catch and remove the aspirated thrombus. AngioVac requires 2 access points for large bore venous sheaths. Commonly, a 26F sheath is placed in either the right common femoral or right internal jugular vein and the reinfusion cannula in a second venous site. Similar technique, as described previously, with the FlowTriever device is required to deliver the AngioVac catheter into the PA. Through the 26F sheath, the AngioVac catheter and obturator are advanced into the PA over a stiff 0.035-in wire, obturator removed, the cannula attached to the tubing of the centrifuge pump, and then the outflow tubing connected to the 18-Freinfusion cannula. When using a right internal jugular approach, the authors have found that the Lunderquist Double-Curve Wire (Cook Medical, Bloomington, Indiana) tends to be easily navigated into the right main PA via a balloon-tipped catheter. This provides excellent support for navigating into the pulmonary trunk or right main PA even in cases of a severely dilated right ventricle. Great care must be taken to manage the distal tip of the wire given the propensity of such a stiff wire to cause perforation of smaller pulmonary arteries. Aspiration is then started and the thrombus is aspirated and captured by filtration canister that is connected proximal to the centrifuge pump. Flow rates of the AngioVac circuit range from 1.5 L/min to 6 L/min as it is a full venovenous extracorporeal membrane oxygenation circuit. When placed in the pulmonary arteries, flows of 1.5 L to 2.5 L are generally targeted. In other circumstances, such as free-floating right-sided clot-in-transit the AngioVac can often successfully run at 4 L to 5 L per minute. The major benefit of this system is the ability to aspirate large volumes of blood and return it filtered to the patient, avoiding significant blood loss.

There are few data on the use of the AngioVac device in PE. There are no large case series or randomized trials, and published experience is limited to case reports and small case series.[16] Like other large bore venous catheters, the major limitations to the AngioVac are large size and inflexibility, which make it difficult to delivery through the tortuosity out into the PA. This can result in damage to the tricuspid valve, perforation, tamponade, and/or bleeding at the access site, especially in patients who also receive thrombolysis. In addition, the AngioVac usually requires a perfusionist to be present to

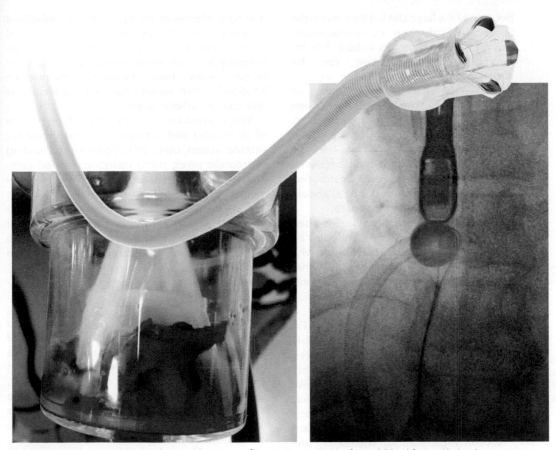

Fig. 5. AngioVac aspiration catheter. (*Courtesy of* AngioDynamics, Latham, NY; with permission.)

assist with the set-up and operation of the system. Given these limitations, it can be difficult to perform emergently for patients with massive PE. Currently, most of the use of the AngioVac catheter is in the treatment of central venous and right atrial thrombi, owing to the difficulty in delivering the stiff catheter to the PA. Some investigators have described direct surgical access into the right ventricule, providing a direct route into the PA and avoiding cardiopulmonary bypass.[17]

ENDPOINTS FOR TREATMENT

Given that none of the techniques described previously, with or without thrombolytic infusion, lead to complete thrombus removal, the following questions about the endpoints of treatment and when to stop the procedure frequently arise:

- Which parameters should be followed to end the procedure: hemodynamic improvement, volume of thrombus removed, number of branches treated,

number of segments with improved perfusion, patient's tolerance of the procedure, and so forth?
- What results constitute a successful procedure both acutely, short term and long term? Are these hemodynamic, anatomic, or functional?

These questions are important for clinical application, for designing research studies, and for examining new technology. Although there are no clear answers to these questions, the following points can give some guidance to that end:

- If a patient is in shock, the goal is to disrupt and aspirate as much of the obstructive clot as possible to allow better lung perfusion. Such cases frequently show complete occlusion in most of the pulmonary segments with central thrombi, and any improvement in forward flow allows for better hemodynamic stability. Once a patient's blood pressure improves and there is demonstration of better forward flow, the procedure can be terminated.

Because of the large clot burden, and in the absence of absolute contraindications, leaving infusion catheters in both PAs for thrombolytic administration can be strongly considered.

- For patients without ongoing shock or whose blood pressure have been stabilized with fluids or low dose pressors, a few factors can be considered as potential endpoints:
  - If there is a clearly occluded lobe(s) with absent perfusion (see **Fig. 3**), restoration of flow to the occluded lobe(s) should signal the end of the procedure.
  - The angiographic thrombus burden should not be used as an endpoint by itself given the poor correlation with hemodynamic significance and that percutaneous thrombectomy is only able to safely remove a small fraction of the clot burden.
  - A significant improvement in the PA pressure should also signal a possible end of the procedure. Care, however, should be exerted to identify other reasons for a drop in PA pressure, like excessive bleeding/blood loss, cardiac or vascular perforation, and damage to the tricuspid valve with resultant severe regurgitation. Measuring the right atrial pressure and the PA oxygen saturation with comparison to the baseline numbers can help rule out such possibilities as reasons for a decrease in PA pressure.
  - If aspiration thrombectomy is performed, how much blood has been lost can influence timing of procedure termination even when desired anatomic or hemodynamic results have not been obtained. Using cell saver technology to reinfuse the filtered blood may help allow for longer procedures.

COMPLICATIONS

The most common complications in PE treatment relate to access site bleeding/hematoma, especially in patients who receive concomitant thrombolytics. Other risks include arrhythmias, cardiac structural damage (pulmonary or tricuspid valve tear in case of large catheters or stiff wires), cardiac tamponade, PA perforation, alveolar hemorrhage/hemoptysis related to reperfusion of infarcted lung tissues, and worsening in hemodynamic or respiratory condition

due to occlusion of PA branches by embolized proximal nonocclusive thrombi. The rate of these complications in percutaneous PA thrombectomy is poorly reported because most published series have included thrombolytic infusion.[8] It also varied based on the technique and size of catheter used.

Ways to reduce complications include the use of ultrasound and micropuncture technique for vascular access, using soft-tipped wires, avoiding hydrophilic wires, using ballooned-tipped catheter to cross the tricuspid valve to avoid entrapment behind a papillary muscle, understanding and defining segmental PA anatomy through adequate angiography prior to advancement of wires and catheters, and stopping early enough in the procedure when acceptable, rather than perfect, results have been achieved.

FUTURE DIRECTIONS

Although the current catheters offer promise to fill an unmet clinical need in the treatment of acute PA, all the current embolectomy catheters have limitations. Understanding the current percutaneous embolectomy catheters, however, can help with speculation on the design of a more optimal embolectomy catheter for the future. Such a catheter would probably require many of the following:

- A 10F to 14F size: the catheter needs to be large enough to remove large thrombus but small enough to track through the tortuous pulmonary anatomy into smaller lobar arteries
- A thrombus retraction mechanism: some form of Fogarty-like catheter retraction is needed to pull the distal clot back into the larger proximal catheter.
- Directionality: the sheath or catheter system needs to change the angle of the bend to better direct catheter into the thrombus.
- Aspiration: aspiration seems the most effective way to remove the clot.
- Ability to return blood: the system will need a mechanism to capture, filter, and return blood removed from the PA so that blood loss is not a limiting factor for thrombectomy.
- Visualization: the system will need the ability to perform angiography through or around the catheter/sheath to guide catheter placement.

In addition to better catheter design, better imaging technology to coregister the pulmonary thrombus and PA anatomy in the angiography suite is needed. Perhaps rotational 3-D invasive angiography with live 3-D fluoroscopy and/or fusion of a 3-D CT angiography overlay with live fluoroscopy can better guide catheter embolectomy in the tortuous pulmonary vasculature. This will require partnership with industry colleagues to better design angiography suites to diagnose and treat PE.

Once technology has improved enough to allow for better thrombus retrieval, randomized trials should be performed to investigate the effect of such technology on both short-term and long-term outcomes, including perceived dyspnea and exercise tolerance after at least 3 months to 6 months. Until then, every effort should be made to include treated patients in prospective registries or trials to have a better understanding of the safety and efficacy of percutaneous PE treatment.

REFERENCES

1. Stein PD, Matta F. Thrombolytic therapy in unstable patients with acute pulmonary embolism: saves lives but underused. Am J Med 2012; 125(5):465–70.

2. Wan S, Quinlan DJ, Agnelli G, et al. Thrombolysis compared with heparin for the initial treatment of pulmonary embolism: a meta-analysis of the randomized controlled trials. Circulation 2004;110(6):744–9.

3. Jaff MR, McMurtry MS, Archer SL, et al. Management of massive and submassive pulmonary embolism, iliofemoral deep vein thrombosis, and chronic thromboembolic pulmonary hypertension: a scientific statement from the American heart association. Circulation 2011;123(16):1788–830.

4. Konstantinides SV, Torbicki A, Agnelli G, et al. 2014 ESC guidelines on the diagnosis and management of acute pulmonary embolism. Eur Heart J 2014; 35(43):3033–69, 3069a–3069k.

5. Tukaye DN, McDaniel M, Liberman H, et al. Percutaneous pulmonary embolus mechanical thrombectomy. JACC Cardiovasc Interv 2017;10(1):94–5.

6. Bloomer TL, El-Hayek GE, McDaniel MC, et al. Safety of catheter-directed thrombolysis for massive and submassive pulmonary embolism: results of a multicenter registry and meta-analysis. Catheter Cardiovasc Interv 2017;89(4):754–60.

7. Jaber WA, Fong PP, Weisz G, et al. Acute pulmonary embolism: with an emphasis on an interventional approach. J Am Coll Cardiol 2016;67(8): 991–1002.

8. Kuo WT, Gould MK, Louie JD, et al. Catheter-directed therapy for the treatment of massive pulmonary embolism: systematic review and meta-analysis of modern techniques. J Vasc Interv Radiol 2009;20(11):1431–40.

9. Cilingiroglu M, Salinger M, Zhao D, et al. Technique of temporary subcutaneous "Figure-of-Eight" sutures to achieve hemostasis after removal of large-caliber femoral venous sheaths. Catheter Cardiovasc Interv 2011;78(1):155–60.

10. Hamid T, Rajagopal R, Pius C, et al. Preclosure of large-sized venous access sites in adults undergoing transcatheter structural interventions. Catheter Cardiovasc Interv 2013;81(4):586–90.

11. Schmitz-Rode T, Janssens U, Duda SH, et al. Massive pulmonary embolism: percutaneous emergency treatment by pigtail rotation catheter. J Am Coll Cardiol 2000;36(2):375–80.

12. Hubbard J, Saad WE, Sabri SS, et al. Rheolytic thrombectomy with or without adjunctive indwelling pharmacolysis in patients presenting with acute pulmonary embolism presenting with right heart strain and/or pulseless electrical activity. Thrombosis 2011;2011:246410.

13. Vecchio S, Vittori G, Chechi T, et al. Percutaneous rheolytic thrombectomy with AngioJet for pulmonary embolism: methods and results in the experience of a high-volume center. G Ital Cardiol (Rome) 2008;9(5):355–63 [in Italian].

14. Kucher N, Windecker S, Banz Y, et al. Percutaneous catheter thrombectomy device for acute pulmonary embolism: in vitro and in vivo testing. Radiology 2005;236(3):852–8.

15. Kumar Bhatia N, Dickert NW, Samady H, et al. The use of hemodynamic support in massive pulmonary embolism. Catheter Cardiovasc Interv 2017;90(3): 516–20.

16. Donaldson CW, Baker JN, Narayan RL, et al. Thrombectomy using suction filtration and venovenous bypass: single center experience with a novel device. Catheter Cardiovasc Interv 2015; 86(2):E81–7.

17. Lumsden AB, Suarez E. Interventional therapy for pulmonary embolism. Methodist Debakey Cardiovasc J 2016;12(4):219–24.

Balloon Pulmonary Angioplasty for Chronic Thromboembolic Pulmonary Hypertension

Ehtisham Mahmud, MD, FSCAI[a],*, Omid Behnamfar, MD[a],
Lawrence Ang, MD[a], Mitul P. Patel, MD[a],
David Poch, MD[b], Nick H. Kim, MD[b]

KEYWORDS

- Chronic thromboembolic pulmonary hypertension (CTEPH)
- Balloon pulmonary angioplasty (BPA) • Pulmonary thromboendarterectomy (PTE)

KEY POINTS

- Chronic thromboembolic pulmonary hypertension (CTEPH), although associated with several risk factors, is a relatively uncommon consequence of acute pulmonary embolism.
- Pulmonary thromboendarterectomy is a potentially curative surgical treatment for CTEPH.
- Medical therapy is limited for surgically inoperable CTEPH and percutaneous balloon pulmonary angioplasty (BPA) is emerging as a new therapeutic option for CTEPH.
- Optimal patient selection, procedural technique and management of complications of BPA are reviewed.
- Early data demonstrate technical feasibility of BPA and short-term success in improving pulmonary hypertension in CTEPH.

Chronic thromboembolic pulmonary hypertension (CTEPH) is a form of precapillary pulmonary hypertension characterized by mean pulmonary artery pressure (mPAP) greater than or equal to 25 mm Hg and pulmonary capillary wedge pressure less than or equal to 15 mm Hg. It results from deposition of thromboembolic material in the pulmonary vascular bed; failure of its dissolution; and formation of a chronic, fibrotic, flow-limiting, organized thrombus. CTEPH is considered a relatively rare outcome following an acute pulmonary embolism,[1–3] occurring in 0.4% to 9.1% of acute pulmonary embolism survivors but in more than 10% of patients with confirmed recurrent pulmonary embolism.[4–9]

However, because most patients with acute pulmonary embolism do not develop CTEPH, several additional factors are also thought to contribute (**Box 1**).[1,2]

CLINICAL PRESENTATION AND DIAGNOSIS

Patients with CTEPH initially present with progressive dyspnea, exercise intolerance, and vague findings on physical examination. With disease progression there is a high risk of developing pulmonary hypertension and right heart failure.[10,11] Ventilation-perfusion (V-Q) lung imaging is recommended as the initial screening

Disclosure: No relevant disclosures.
[a] Division of Cardiovascular Medicine, Sulpizio Cardiovascular Center, University of California, San Diego, 9434 Medical Center Drive, La Jolla, CA 92037, USA; [b] Division of Pulmonary and Critical Care Medicine, Sulpizio Cardiovascular Center, University of California, San Diego, 9434 Medical Center Drive, La Jolla, CA 92037, USA
* Corresponding author.
E-mail address: emahmud@ucsd.edu

Intervent Cardiol Clin 7 (2018) 103–117
https://doi.org/10.1016/j.iccl.2017.09.003
2211-7458/18/© 2017 Elsevier Inc. All rights reserved.

Acute pulmonary embolism

Multiple pulmonary embolic events

Large perfusion defect

Higher pulmonary artery pressure at time of diagnosis

Idiopathic (unprovoked) presentation

Hemostatic risk factors

Elevated factor VIII, von Willebrand factor, type 1 plasminogen activator inhibitor

Abnormal fibrinogen structure

Non–type-O blood groups

Elevated lipoprotein(a)

Associated medical conditions

Splenectomy

Ventriculoatrial shunt

Infected intravenous catheters or devices

Chronic inflammatory disorders

Antiphospholipid antibodies and lupus anticoagulant

Hypothyroidism

Cancer

test for evaluating patients with suspected CTEPH (**Fig. 1**).[3,10,11] Images demonstrate lobar-level or segmental-level mismatched perfusion defects in proximal vessel disease, or mottled and patchy perfusion defects in the lung periphery in distal subsegmental disease (**Fig. 2**).[12,13] V-Q scan findings suggesting CTEPH such as these are nonspecific and the diagnosis must be confirmed by additional imaging modalities, including computed tomographic pulmonary angiography, MRI, and/or invasive pulmonary angiography.[14,15]

INVASIVE PULMONARY ANGIOGRAPHY AND RIGHT HEART CATHETERIZATION

Catheter-based pulmonary angiography has been considered the gold standard imaging in the evaluation of CTEPH. When combined with right heart catheterization, it can confirm the presence of pulmonary thromboembolic disease and exclude other possible diagnoses, evaluate effects on pulmonary artery pressure and right heart function, and determine surgical accessibility of the disease.[16,17] Because diagnostic angiography is crucial for identifying high-grade proximal thromboembolic pulmonary disease warranting surgical resection or interventional treatment, image optimization is critically important.

The right internal jugular vein allows for right heart catheterization and bilateral pulmonary

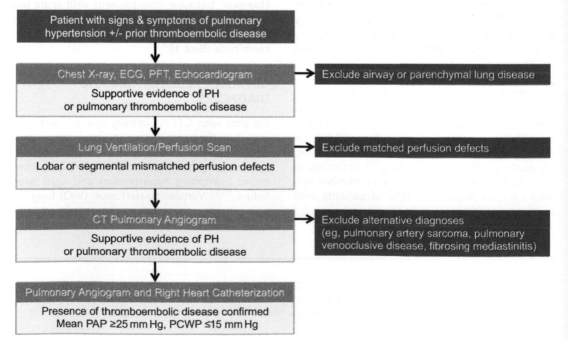

Fig. 1. Diagnostic workup of chronic thromboembolic pulmonary hypertension. CT, computed tomography; ECG, electrocardiogram; PAP, pulmonary artery pressure; PCWP, pulmonary capillary wedge pressure; X-ray, radiograph.

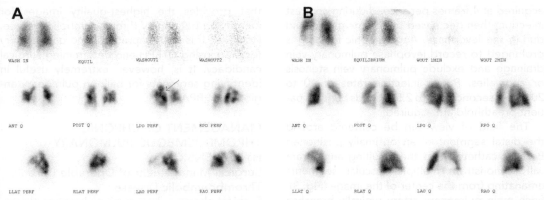

Fig. 2. Comparison of abnormal lung ventilation-perfusion images. (*A*) CTEPH with multiple bilateral perfusion defects as opposed to (*B*), a proximal left pulmonary artery mass.

artery angiography in the most expedient manner using standard balloon-tipped, flow-directed catheters. Vascular ultrasound imaging is used to evaluate the caliber, patency, and collapsibility of the jugular vein before venipuncture. Right heart catheterization with hemodynamic and cardiac output measurements using a standard balloon-tipped Swan-Ganz thermodilution pulmonary artery catheter (Edwards, Irvine, CA, USA) is routinely performed before pulmonary angiography. Most patients presenting for this procedure are in a compensated low-cardiac output state and can proceed immediately from right heart catheterization to selective pulmonary angiography.

The standard Berman catheter (Teleflex, Wayne, PA, USA), is well-suited for pulmonary angiography. The Berman catheter is a balloon-tipped, end-capped, pressure-rated catheter that is safely and easily advanced through the right heart and into the pulmonary artery. The end cap protects the distal pulmonary vasculature from iatrogenic injury during high-pressure injections. Multiple fenestrations along the catheter tip allow for pressure diffusion and rapid contrast egress. The flow-directed, preshaped Berman catheter usually tracks into the right pulmonary artery with ease. Catheter redirection from the main pulmonary artery trunk to the left branch is easily performed by straightening the catheter tip (by inserting the stiff end of any 0.035-inch wire into the central lumen and abutting the distal cap), inflating the distal balloon, and advancing the catheter or wire assembly during a patient's deep breathhold. Once the catheter clearly enters the proximal left pulmonary artery, the wire can be removed and the catheter advanced more distally via flow-direction alone. Advancement of the relatively stiff Berman catheter through the right heart is more difficult when performed from the

femoral vein approach and should be avoided. Other catheter options such as standard Swan-Ganz, pigtail, Omni Flush (Angiodynamics, Latham, NY, USA), or preshaped end-hole catheters have previously been used for pulmonary angiography but have various limitations.

Once the Berman catheter is advanced close to pulmonary capillary wedge position in the lung of interest, the distal balloon is deflated and central lumen flushed. During a patient's breathhold, the catheter position is optimized to allow for small movement of the catheter tip with each heart beat (~1 cm of migration during each beat). The optimal position for the Berman tip is within the proximal lower lobar artery, which allows for simultaneous opacification of the middle and lower lung zones, quickly followed by backfilling of upper lobe vessels. The vasculature of these middle and lower lung zones typically bear greater disease burden and are of higher clinical interest during angiography.

Biplane subtraction pulmonary angiography requires attention to (1) patient positioning, (2) flat detector angulation, (3) collimation, and (4) imaging system settings. Once the Berman catheter is positioned within the pulmonary artery of interest, the patient raises and maintains both arms above shoulder level (usually with the patient's hands clasped behind the head) to limit humeral bone interference and motion artifact. When obtaining right pulmonary angiograms, the frontal and lateral flat detectors are kept in straight anterior-posterior (AP) and left lateral (or left anterior oblique [LAO] 90°) views, respectively. Left pulmonary angiograms can be performed in straight AP and left lateral views. Rotation of views 20° leftward (to LAO 20° and LAO 110°, respectively) is traditionally performed to decrease overlap of the mediastinum and left lung, but is not necessary with digital subtraction angiography. Frontal and lateral angiograms are acquired at 4 frames per second during contrast injection, then decreased to 1 frame per second during the levophase. Angiographic imaging is prolonged to record levophase pulmonary vein drainage and exclude pulmonary vein stenosis or anomalies. Power injection rates of 10 to 20 cc per second for 2 to 2.5 seconds during a patient breathhold are acquired.

The field of view can be centered around the distal segment of an optimally positioned Berman catheter, and the resulting angiogram will demonstrate multiple vascular segments emanating from the center of the image (**Fig. 3**). Each main pulmonary artery typically branches into 10 different segments. The superior lobar artery supplies the upper lobe and branches into apical (A1), posterior (A2), and anterior (A3) segments. Proximal branches emanating from the ongoing interlobar artery course anteriorly to the lateral (A4) and medial (A5) regions of the middle or lingular lobe, and posteriorly to the superior segment of the lower lobe (A6). The ongoing basal trunk branches into to the medial basal (A7), anterior basal (A8), lateral basal (A9) and posterior basal (A10) segments.

Characteristic pulmonary angiographic findings suggestive of CTEPH include webs or bands, intimal irregularities, pouch defects, abrupt vascular narrowing, and complete obstruction of pulmonary arteries[18] (**Fig. 4**). Subselective invasive angiography of individual pulmonary artery segments is a feasible procedure that provides the highest-quality images for identifying pulmonary thromboembolic disease. However, it is both impractical and unnecessary for diagnosing CTEPH and determining surgical candidacy. It is, however, extremely useful in identifying segments for balloon pulmonary angioplasty (BPA).

MANAGEMENT OF CHRONIC THROMBOEMBOLIC PULMONARY HYPERTENSION
Surgical Management of Operable Chronic Thromboembolic Disease
Surgical therapy, known as pulmonary thromboendarterectomy (PTE) or pulmonary endarterectomy, is performed via median sternotomy and requires cardiopulmonary bypass and complete circulatory arrest with deep hypothermia to remove thromboembolic material from the pulmonary vasculature.[19] Historically accepted indications for PTE were a mPAP greater than 30 mm Hg, pulmonary vascular resistance (PVR) greater than 300 dyne-sec-cm^{-5}, and New York Heart Association functional classification of III-IV.[20,21] However, currently, it is indicated for symptomatic disease. Operability assessment accounts for surgical accessibility, presence of hemodynamic or ventilatory impairments, and evaluation of underlying comorbidities prohibiting PTE.[22] Perioperative mortality is increased with markedly elevated preoperative PVR greater than 1000 dyne-sec-cm^{-5}, and to an

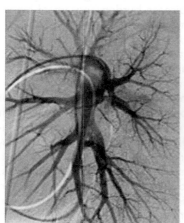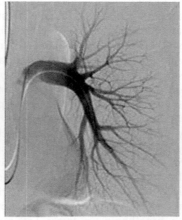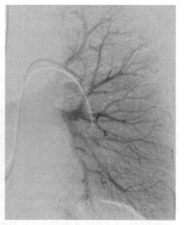

Fig. 3. Selective left pulmonary angiogram. This high-quality pulmonary angiogram shows initial Berman catheter tip position within a left lower lobe pulmonary artery segment. There is complete, dense opacification of the entire left pulmonary artery tree, with backfilling of left upper lobe segments and minimal contrast spillover into the contralateral lung. Insignificant motion artifact, especially of the diaphragm and lower lung zone, is observed during digital subtraction angiography. The resulting image clearly visualizes the course and character of the left pulmonary artery, segments, and subsegments in lateral (*left*) and frontal (*center*) views, as well as pulmonary vein drainage into the left atrium (*right*).

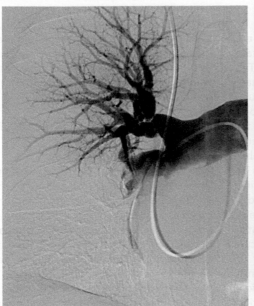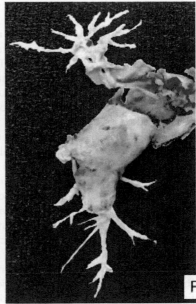

Fig. 4. Selective right pulmonary angiogram and surgically resected specimen of a CTEPH patient with proximal disease. Characteristic findings include band formation, segmental webs, lining thrombus, abrupt vessel tapering, and vessel occlusion (*left*). Surgically resected specimen reveals extent of disease with the proximally occluded right lower lobe and evidence of upper lobe disease on angiography (*right*).

even greater extent with residual pulmonary hypertension following PTE, which can be seen in up to 35% of patients undergoing surgery.[23–26] However, severity of preoperative PVR and the degree of pulmonary hypertension should not be considered a contraindication to surgical intervention because these patients may ultimately benefit from surgery.[24,27] Patients undergoing PTE may experience various complications similar to other cardiothoracic surgical procedures, such as arrhythmias, pericardial or pleural effusions, atelectasis, wound infection, and delirium. Notably, reperfusion pulmonary edema (RPE), a type of noncardiogenic high-permeability pulmonary edema occurs in 9.6% of patients after PTE and can present with mild postoperative hypoxemia to severe hemorrhagic pulmonary edema.[28,29] The risk of RPE is increased in patients with high preoperative and persistent post-PTE pulmonary hypertension.[30]

Medical Therapy for Chronic Thromboembolic Pulmonary Hypertension
Pulmonary hypertension–directed targeted medical therapy as an alternative option for the treatment of CTEPH is indicated in those with inoperable disease, and for patients having experienced suboptimal hemodynamic and functional results following PTE surgery. Currently, riociguat is the only therapy approved

for this indication based on the results of the CHEST-1 study.[31,32] However, even before the approval of riociguat, CTEPH patients were often treated with therapies approved for pulmonary arterial hypertension (PAH).[33] However, the subgroup of PTE patients pretreated with PAH therapies had no significant advantage compared with those without medical therapy. Instead, the medically treated group had a significant time delay in referral for surgery compared with the rest. Accordingly, treatment guidelines emphasize the importance of operability evaluation by an experienced CTEPH team as the first step before reaching for medical therapy.[34]

Interventional Treatment of Chronic Thromboembolic Pulmonary Hypertension
BPA, also known as percutaneous transluminal pulmonary angioplasty, is a procedure initially proposed for the treatment of congenital pulmonary artery stenosis in younger patients.[35,36] The initial feasibility study describing the beneficial effects of BPA as an alternative treatment of selected patients with inoperable CTEPH was reported almost 2 decades ago,[37,38] but the approach was abandoned due to the frequency of major complications. However, over the past 5 years, the procedure has undergone refinement with promising feasibility data from various centers around the world.

Patient Selection for Balloon Pulmonary Angioplasty

Patient selection criteria for treatment are among the most controversial and least standardized aspects of using BPA for CTEPH. The authors recommend that a multidisciplinary team approach consisting of pulmonary vascular medicine specialists, interventional cardiologists, and PTE surgical experts be in place for evaluating and identifying appropriate patients with CTEPH for BPA (Fig. 5). Surgical inoperability is a contentious issue and highly depends on local surgical expertise, patient comorbidities, proximal versus distal pulmonary segmental disease, and patient preference.[11] BPA has been performed in most patients for symptomatic, inoperable CTEPH[39–46] or for persistent or recurrent pulmonary hypertension following PTE.[47–49] Rescue BPA has also been reported as a transitional or bridging treatment option in rapidly deteriorating CTEPH patients for stabilization before PTE.[48,49] BPA can also be combined with PTE in selected CTEPH patients with surgically accessible disease for 1 lung and inoperable disease affecting the contralateral lung.[50] In general, lobar and proximal segmental disease is better suited for surgical resection, whereas distal segmental and subsegmental disease is more appropriate for BPA.

APPROACH TO BALLOON PULMONARY ANGIOPLASTY

General Treatment Strategy

Although there is no consistent and agreed on technique for the performance of BPA, this article describes the approach the authors have taken at UC San Diego (Box 2). A complete treatment course usually involves 4 to 6 separate BPA procedures, spaced apart by 3 to 7 days, and concluded by 1 final treatment in each lung. Target vessels are identified based on noninvasive lung perfusion scans with the goal to revascularize the areas with the largest perfusion defects. Intermittent perfusion scanning is

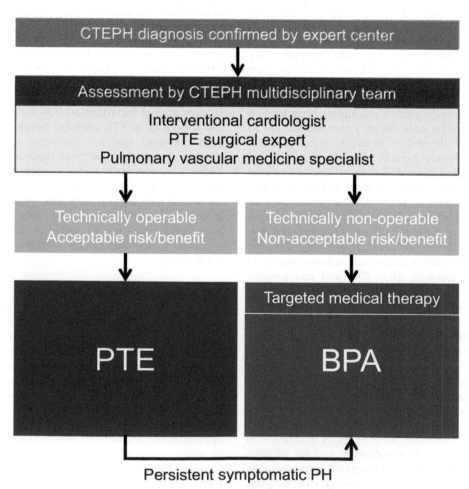

Fig. 5. Suggested CTEPH treatment algorithm by a multidisciplinary team.

Box 2
Stepwise approach to balloon pulmonary angioplasty

Overall treatment plan

- Four to 6 separate BPA sessions
- Baseline pulmonary angiogram plus or minus computed tomography angiogram
- Baseline and intermittent perfusion scanning
- Baseline and intermittent clinical evaluation
- Baseline and intermittent 6-minute walk testing
- Treatment concluded with 1 BPA procedure in each lung

Individual BPA procedure steps

1. Identify target lung region with largest defect on most recent perfusion scan.
2. Ultrasound-guided right (or left) femoral vein access, 9-French sheath placement.
3. Right heart catheterization and hemodynamic measurement within target lung.
4. Pulmonary artery catheter removed over guidewire.
5. 6-French 90-cm sheath advanced over wire into target lung pulmonary artery.
6. Anticoagulation using intravenous (IV) unfractionated heparin (goal ACT 200–250 seconds).
7. 6-French 110-cm Judkins right or multipurpose guide catheter advanced over stiff, angled Glidewire into target lung region.
8. Guide catheter is used to selectively engage pulmonary artery segments of interest.
9. Segmental pulmonary angiography is performed with deep breathholds and injection of 1:1 diluted contrast.
10. Atraumatic, workhorse 0.014-inch guidewire, supported by 2.0-mm rapid exchange balloon catheter, is used to cross target lesions. Recommend avoiding specialty wires with higher perforation risk.
11. Pd/Pa measurements during free breathing or deep breathhold can be measured. Recommend microcatheter based pressure measurements for easy and repeated use during BPA. Guidewires are often deformed and exchanged during BPA procedures.
12. Serial balloon inflation using 2.0 to 4.0 mm semicompliant and noncompliant balloons. Recommend serial dilations and undersizing balloons to avoid vessel perforation or rupture.
13. Repeat above steps for treatment of other diseased segments of interest.
14. Procedure conclusion when 3 to 5 diseased segments are treated during an initial session, 400 mL IV contrast is administered, and/or 2 Gy exposure reached.
15. Manual sheath removal once activated clotting time less than 180 seconds.

---

repeated to observe overall changes in lung perfusion from baseline and reprioritize diseased regions. Six-minute walk tests are performed at baseline and repeated at intervals to follow the clinical response to treatment. Right heart catheterization and hemodynamic measurements before each BPA procedure monitor the cumulative effect of treatment on cardiopulmonary hemodynamics. Any single procedure is limited to no more than 2 Gy of radiation exposure and/or 400 mL of administered contrast.

Vascular Access
Before each BPA procedure, femoral vein access with placement of a 9-French vascular introducer sheath is achieved using ultrasound guidance.

The femoral vein is preferred to the internal jugular or brachial veins as a conduit for BPA to optimize operator ease-of-use and limit radiation exposure. Following right heart catheterization, a single-lumen wedge catheter is directed into the target lung and exchanged over an 0.035-in guidewire for a 90-cm 6-French sheath that is advanced beyond the common pulmonary artery segment. Through this second sheath, a 6-French preshaped guide catheter can be advanced over a guidewire and directed for selective pulmonary artery angiography and intervention.

Segmental Pulmonary Angiography
A 6-French guide catheter is carefully advanced through the long pulmonary artery sheath and

over a stiff angled Glidewire (Terumo, Tokyo, Japan) into the pulmonary lobe of interest. Most procedures are performed using Judkins Right and Multipurpose catheter shapes. The Extra Backup (EBU) guide catheter shapes are reserved for the lingual and occasionally middle lobe segments. Careful guide catheter manipulation is performed to selectively engage different pulmonary artery segments. Target vessel evaluation by selective segmental pulmonary artery angiograms before and during the BPA procedure provides valuable information on vessel size, target lesion characteristics, distal pulmonary artery flow, and pulmonary venous drainage in response to therapy. These angiograms are performed following selective guide catheter engagement and injection of 1:1 saline diluted contrast. Angiograms are acquired during deep breathholds at 7.5 to 15 frames per second without digital subtraction. Angiograms of higher frame rate and quality can help with detailed lesion characterization but are generally not necessary. Simultaneous biplane angiography also offers more imaging data, especially helpful for tortuous or overlapping vessels, but the authors have exclusively shifted to single-plane angiography to minimize patient radiation dose and operator exposure.

Target Lesion Characterization

Traditional characterization of lesions based on angiography have remained essentially unchanged since their initial description. Characteristic pulmonary angiographic findings suggestive of CTEPH include webs or bands, intimal irregularities, pouch defects, abrupt vascular narrowing, and complete obstruction of pulmonary arteries.[18] However, contemporary imaging modalities, including intravascular ultrasound (IVUS), optical coherence tomography (OCT), and cone beam computed tomography (CBCT) have been used in CTEPH for adjunctive lesion characterization and BPA guidance.[39,41,51,52]

A study with 9 prospectively enrolled distal CTEPH subjects demonstrated OCT to be superior to IVUS during the BPA procedure in detecting the chronic thromboembolic lesion, providing a more accurate measurement of luminal diameter and optimizing procedural success in properly dilating the distal pulmonary arteries with long thrombus-occluded lesions.[53] IVUS-Virtual Histology (IVUS-VH) uses reflected IVUS signals on the arterial wall to create a color-coded image and allow analysis of intraarterial lesion composition.[54] In a study using IVUS-VH, in vivo characterization of target

lesions in CTEPH before and after BPA showed that fibrous tissue, represented by green color coding, was most compressible, whereas the red and white coded areas representing necrotic core and dense calcium, respectively, were least responsive to angioplasty.[55]

Webs and slit-like lesions in distal segments are usually the main targets for the BPA procedure. More severely obstructed lesions may also be approached provided antegrade or collateral flow past the lesion is confirmed.[52] Sugiyama and colleagues[56] evaluated the usefulness of CBCT in assessment of organized thrombus in more distal pulmonary artery segments in CTEPH and suggested a new classification of distal lesions (type 1: webs, type 2: web and slits, type 3: slits, and type 4: narrowing or complete occlusion). In their report, the combination of webs and slits were shown to be the most common type of lesions found in distal segments by CBCT that are not clearly visible with other standard imaging techniques.[56] However, at the authors' center and in our experience, the primary anatomic imaging modality to identify optimal targets for BPA remains segmental pulmonary angiography.

Pulmonary Artery Intervention

Techniques to perform BPA have undergone significant modification since initial reports. Contemporary BPA aims to disrupt organized, flow-limiting obstructions and improve pulmonary vascular blood flow while avoiding complications (**Fig. 6**). Unlike coronary artery and peripheral vascular interventions in which symptomatic relief can be experienced after revascularization of a single vessel, clinical improvement following BPA is typically observed after revascularization of multiple diseased segments and regions. Aggressive intervention of individual lesions with increased risk of vascular injury can be counterproductive to the overall treatment strategy. We generally treat 1 to 2 pulmonary lobes in the same lung during any single BPA procedure.

To help avoid vascular injury, 0.014-in workhouse guidewires with soft, atraumatic, spring-coil tips are used for BPA. Almost all of our BPA procedures are performed using the Hi-Torque Balanced Middle Weight wire (Abbott Vascular, Abbott Park, IL, USA). Even when treating occluded vessels, we favor using an atraumatic wire in conjunction with catheter support and judicious use of antegrade wire escalation with increased guidewire tip stiffness. However, we use caution in utilization of hydrophilic guidewires because early experience for

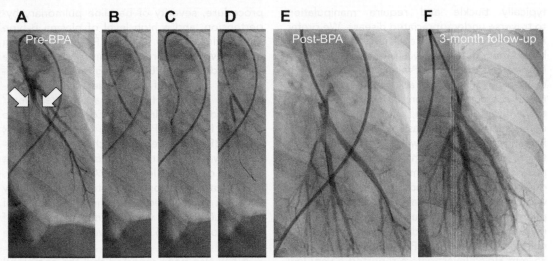

Fig. 6. BPA of the left lower lobe. BPA of a severely-diseased left A10 (*left arrow*) and left A9 (*right arrow*) segments (*A*). Serial balloon dilation was performed (*B, C*) with final kissing balloon inflation using noncompliant 3.0-mm (A10) and 3.5-mm (A9) diameter balloons (*D*). Improved residual stenosis and distal vessel runoff was observed immediately following intervention (*E*) and vessel remodeling observed at 3-month follow-up (*F*).

us and others suggests increased risk of vascular injury and pulmonary hemorrhage using polymer jacketed guidewires.[46] Unfractionated heparin is administered for procedural anticoagulation with an activated clotting time (ACT) goal of 200 to 250 seconds.

Small-diameter, compliant balloons are selected for initial balloon angioplasty to help determine vessel diameter and lesion response before larger balloons are used. Most distal pulmonary vascular lesions can be initially treated using 2.0 mm diameter balloons. Proximal segment angioplasty is performed with sequential balloon inflations using larger-diameter, noncompliant balloons typically ranging between 2.5 to 4.0 mm, and rarely up to 5.0 mm. Balloons with smaller diameters than the target vessel are preferred to preserve the pulmonary arterial architecture and minimize the risk of dissection, perforation, or rupture.[40]

In some instances, special techniques are considered when target lesion recoil is observed despite serial balloon inflations and appropriate balloon sizing. First, multiple prolonged balloon inflations up to 3 minutes in duration are attempted. Next, lesion modification using specialty devices such as the Chocolate (TriReme Medical LLC, Pleasanton, CA, USA) and AngioSculpt (Spectranetics Corp, Colorado Springs, CO, USA) balloon catheters can be attempted with prolonged balloon inflation. More aggressive approaches using cutting balloons or atherectomy catheters increase risk of vessel injury and

should be avoided. Deployment of covered stents for catastrophic rupture is possible. Although data for long-term pulmonary artery patency following BPA are limited, restenosis is considered uncommon[41] and stenting to prevent restenosis after balloon angioplasty is not recommended, especially because there is significant pulmonary vascular mobility during the respiratory phase.[39–41]

Attention to procedural safety during BPA is further emphasized by avoiding aggressive techniques during initial treatment sessions, especially in the presence of high-grade obstructions or occlusions, and elevated baseline pulmonary artery pressure ($\geq$ mPAP 35 mm Hg) due to higher risk of RPE and hemoptysis. Treatment of 1 to 2 lobes of a single lung (3–5 segments) is recommended per session to decrease this risk and limit both contrast and radiation exposure.[39–41] Initial revascularization of occluded segments aims to restore distal blood flow, improve hemodynamics, and provide a conduit for future repeat and perhaps more aggressive intervention.

Functional Assessment

Prediction of obstructive pulmonary artery disease is difficult by angiography alone and relatively normal-appearing vessels within pulmonary segments underperfused by noninvasive imaging warrant intravascular functional assessment. In cases of uncertainty, advancing a guidewire into the vessel and measuring distal vessel pressure is useful. The tip of the guidewire will typically buckle and require manipulation to traverse underappreciated disease. We prefer measuring distal pressure using a microcatheter-based manometer (Navvus MicroCatheter, Acist Medical Systems, Eden Prairie, MN, USA), which can be advanced over any guidewire and can reveal pressure reduction during diastole alone, the entire cardiac cycle, or complete pressure dampening with increasingly severe disease. Pressure measurement will also fluctuate during the respiratory cycle. There is no standardized protocol for pressure measurement or subsequent therapy. In 1 study, the BPA procedure was continued with the aim of achieving a distal pulmonary artery pressure to proximal pulmonary artery pressure (Pd/Pa) greater than 0.80 unless the baseline mPAP was greater than 35 mm Hg.[57] Investigators reported a very low rate of procedure-related adverse events using this strategy and were able to avoid RPE in most patients. The authors' strategy has been to use a Pd/Pa ratio for treatment guidance with values less than 0.75 prompting additional balloon dilation (larger balloons, higher pressures, or scoring balloons or guidewires). Any improvement in postangioplasty Pd/Pa is sufficient to conclude treatment within the target vessel because frequently during follow-up hemodynamic assessment, the pressure gradients show further improvement either via thrombus resolution or increased flow in the newly revascularized pulmonary segment. Interval noninvasive perfusion scans between therapy sessions are also useful to evaluate perfusion within treated segments and support repeat intervention for areas with persistent hypoperfusion.

Adverse events during balloon pulmonary angioplasty

The procedural outcomes of BPA largely depend on appropriate patient selection, operator expertise, and incorporation of new devices and techniques used in coronary interventions to the pulmonary vasculature. The overall result and rate of complications varies among the centers with different levels of proficiency and volume of patients treated. In recent series, BPA periprocedural mortality ranged from 0% to 10%.[39–46]

The 2 most common complications of BPA include RPE and pulmonary vascular injury with rare episodes of vessel perforation or rupture. Despite the advances and improvement of the procedure, RPE remains a frequent complication of BPA with an incidence as high as 53% to 60% in some studies.[40,41] Several factors associated with RPE following BPA include first

procedure, severity of baseline pulmonary hypertension, and a high level of plasma B-type natriuretic peptide.[38,40] CTEPH patients with underdeveloped bronchial arteries are more likely to develop RPE following the BPA procedure.[58] In a study of 150 consecutive BPA procedures in CTEPH, Inami and colleagues[59] proposed the Pulmonary Edema Predictive Scoring Index (PEPSI), as a product of PVR before BPA and the sum of changes in pulmonary flow grades with the procedure, to predict the risk of RPE following BPA. In their study, PEPSI was the strongest factor, among study variables, correlated with the occurrence of RPE ($P<.0001$) and was a marker of the risk of RPE (cutoff value 35.4, negative predictive value 92.3%).

It has also been reported that the combined approach of pressure wire guidance to measure gradients across stenosis and the PEPSI score might be useful in reducing the risk of RPE and vascular complications.[57] This approach to finishing each BPA session using the PEPSI with the goal of scores less than 35.4 and the guidance of pressure wire to achieve a distal mean pulmonary arterial pressure less than 35 mm Hg in each target lesion, resulted in similar hemodynamic improvements as BPA without this guidance, but associated with fewer numbers of BPA procedures and treated target lesions, and absence of RPE.[57] The combined approach of balloon angioplasty with undersized balloons and reduced number of treated vessels per session might be an effective tool in reducing the risk of developing RPE. However, no definitive data exist to support this approach.

Pulmonary artery perforation or rupture is a serious complication of BPA and is reported in 0% to 7% of procedures in recent studies.[40–42,60] Some measures suggested to decrease the risk of pulmonary artery perforation include proper wire positioning, knuckle-wire technique, appropriate balloon sizing, and avoidance of occluded segments without distal flow.[52] Noninvasive positive-pressure ventilation with supplemental oxygen and, in more severe situations, mechanical ventilation and extracorporeal membrane oxygenation (ECMO), should be considered as the first therapeutic strategy for severe lung injury or vascular rupture following BPA to maintain oxygenation and preserve blood pressure.[61] Immediate balloon tamponade of the perforated or ruptured vessel, cessation, or reversal of anticoagulation, covered stent implantation, Gelfoam injection, and transcatheter coil embolization are suggested bailout techniques with probable benefits in these situations (**Box 3**).[41,61]

Box 3
Management of pulmonary vascular injury during balloon pulmonary angioplasty

1. Immediate balloon tamponade of the injured vessel.
2. Oxygenation management, including oropharyngeal suctioning, supplemental oxygen, noninvasive positive pressure ventilation (mechanical ventilation and ECMO in respiratory failure).
3. Cessation or reversal of anticoagulation.
4. Repeat prolonged balloon tamponade as necessary.
5. For persistent pulmonary hemorrhage consider bailout transcatheter coil embolization, covered stent implantation, and/or Gelfoam or adipose injection.

Clinical outcomes of balloon pulmonary angioplasty

Although the available data on long-term outcomes of BPA in CTEPH are limited (Table 1), in the short-term, the procedure is associated with improvements in cardiopulmonary hemodynamics, pulmonary perfusion, exercise tolerance, World Health Organization functional class, and 6-minute walk distance.[39,41–44,62] Hemodynamic improvements, such as decrease in mPAP and PVR, is proportional to the number of treated vessels.[40,44] Importantly, pulmonary hypertension does not resolve immediately during or following a BPA session, and it can take a few weeks to observe the positive impacts of the procedure.[41,63] Studies have shown improvement in the quality of life and symptom resolution disproportionate to the degree of reduction in pulmonary hypertension.[64] Although limited to a single retrospective series, recent longer term

follow-up shows persistence of hemodynamic benefit (reduction in PVR and pulmonary artery pressure) of the BPA procedure at a median of 2.8 years after procedural completion.[45]

Improvement in right ventricular function has been demonstrated by transthoracic echocardiography using speckle-tracking, 3-dimensional echocardiography, and cardiovascular MRI before and after BPA.[60,65,66] Improved hemodynamics after BPA may lead to RV reverse remodeling, improved systolic function, and reduced subclinical myocardial injury with reduced high-sensitivity troponin T level.[67] Secondary BPA effect on renal function was evaluated in a recent study including 46 CTEPH subjects with or without impaired baseline renal function.[68] A statistically significant improvement of estimated glomerular filtration rate in the impaired renal function group after final BPA session was reported (47.0 vs 51.5 mL/min/1.73 m^2; $P = .018$). This result was consistent with a previous report on the positive effect of BPA on renal function due to severe right heart failure secondary to CTEPH.[69] A study of 9 CTEPH patients with gradually deteriorated PVR at 4.1 (2.7–7.9) years after PTE, reported significant improvement in PVR of 4.2 (2.8–4.8) wood units ($P<.05$) at 1.9 (1.3–3.3) years after subsequent BPA procedures.[47] Safety and efficacy of the procedure has also been demonstrated in elderly patients (age ≥65 years) compared with younger patients, with similar change of hemodynamics, rate of periprocedural complications, length of intensive care unit and in-hospital stay, and all-cause mortality.[70]

Future directions for balloon pulmonary angioplasty

The currently available data from multiple centers around the world indicate the clinical

Table 1
Balloon pulmonary angioplasty studies reporting long-term outcomes

First Author, Year Published	Subjects (Country)	Procedures (Total)	Procedures/ Patient	Long-Term Survival
Feinstein et al,[38] 2001	18 (USA)	47	2.6	89% at 34.2 mo
Mizoguchi et al,[41] 2012	68 (Japan)	255	3.8	97% at 2.2 ± 1.4 y
Sugimura et al,[39] 2012	12 (Japan)	NA	5	100% at 12 mo
Andreassen et al,[42] 2013	20 (Norway)	73	3.7	85% at 51 mo
Yanagisawa et al,[70] 2014	70 (Japan)	257	4 (age <65 y)	100% (<65 y)
			3 (age ≥65 y)	96.8% (≥65 y) at 12 mo
Shimura et al,[47] 2015	110 (Japan)	423	3.8	100% at 1.97 y
Inami et al,[45] 2016	170 (Japan)	649	3.8	97.6% at 2.8 y

feasibility of BPA for the treatment of CTEPH. Among the issues to address are the following:

- Development of CTEPH teams
- Optimal standardized technique
- Development of dedicated interventional equipment
- Appropriate training standards
- Multicenter evaluation with objective adjudication for acute success
- Evaluation of long term outcomes
- Randomized clinical trial of BPA versus medical therapy for inoperable CTEPH
- Randomized clinical trial of BPA versus PTE for segmental disease in CTEPH.

SUMMARY

There have been remarkable improvements in treatment options for CTEPH patients over the past decade. PTE remains the only definitive and potentially curative therapy, whereas medical therapy provides less promising results than surgery and is limited to those not responsive to PTE, inoperable patients, or as a bridge to surgery in high-risk patients. The BPA procedure with introduction of new techniques and technologies is a practical alternative to PTE for select CTEPH patients not amenable to surgery. Despite all the advances in BPA, there is no standard technique to be globally adopted and patient selection remains a significant challenge. There are no clear data on long-term benefits and prognosis of BPA, which highlights the need for future registries with the ultimate goal of randomized controlled trials to determine the safety and efficacy of the procedure.

Due to these uncertainties, and with evolving management approaches, CTEPH patients should be referred to an advanced center experienced in the evaluation and care of this unique patient population. A comprehensive review by a multidisciplinary team to assess operability and to determine the most appropriate mode of therapy remains the optimal treatment strategy.

REFERENCES

1. Lang IM, Pesavento R, Bonderman D, et al. Risk factors and basic mechanisms of chronic thromboembolic pulmonary hypertension: a current understanding. Eur Respir J 2013;41(2):462–8.
2. Kim NH, Lang IM. Risk factors for chronic thromboembolic pulmonary hypertension. Eur Respir Rev 2012;21:27–31.
3. Galie N, Hoeper MM, Humbert M, et al. Guidelines for the diagnosis and treatment of pulmonary hypertension: the Task Force for the Diagnosis and Treatment of Pulmonary Hypertension of the European Society of Cardiology (ESC) and the European Respiratory Society (ERS), endorsed by the International Society of Heart and Lung Transplantation (ISHLT). Eur Heart J 2009;30(20):2493–537.
4. Pengo V, Lensing AW, Prins MH, et al. Incidence of chronic thromboembolic pulmonary hypertension after pulmonary embolism. N Engl J Med 2004; 350(22):2257–64.
5. Becattini C, Agnelli G, Pesavento R, et al. Incidence of chronic thromboembolic pulmonary hypertension after a first episode of pulmonary embolism. Chest 2006;130(1):172–5.
6. Dentali F, Donadini M, Gianni M, et al. Incidence of chronic pulmonary hypertension in patients with previous pulmonary embolism. Thromb Res 2009; 124(3):256–8.
7. Gall H, Hoeper MM, Richter MJ, et al. An epidemiological analysis of the burden of chronic thromboembolic pulmonary hypertension in the USA, Europe and Japan. Eur Respir Rev 2017; 26:160121.
8. Korkmaz A, Ozlu T, Ozsu S, et al. Long-term outcomes in acute pulmonary thromboembolism: the incidence of chronic thromboembolic pulmonary hypertension and associated risk factors. Clin Appl Thromb Hemost 2012;18(3):281–8.
9. Guerin L, Couturaud F, Parent F, et al. Prevalence of chronic thromboembolic pulmonary hypertension after acute pulmonary embolism. Prevalence of CTEPH after pulmonary embolism. Thromb Haemost 2014;112(3):598–605.
10. Fedullo PF, Auger WR, Kerr KM, et al. Chronic thromboembolic pulmonary hypertension. N Engl J Med 2001;345(20):1465–72.
11. Kim NH, Delcroix M, Jenkins DP, et al. Chronic thromboembolic pulmonary hypertension. J Am Coll Cardiol 2013;62(25 Suppl):D92–9.
12. Lisbona R, Kreisman H, Novales-Diaz J, et al. Perfusion lung scanning: differentiation of primary from thromboembolic pulmonary hypertension. AJR Am J Roentgenol 1985;144(1):27–30.
13. Powe JE, Palevsky HI, McCarthy KE, et al. Pulmonary arterial hypertension: value of perfusion scintigraphy. Radiology 1987;164(3):727–30.
14. Tunariu N, Gibbs SJ, Win Z, et al. Ventilation-perfusion scintigraphy is more sensitive than multidetector CTPA in detecting chronic thromboembolic pulmonary disease as a treatable cause of pulmonary hypertension. J Nucl Med 2007;48(5): 680–4.
15. Ryan KL, Fedullo PF, Davis GB, et al. Perfusion scan findings understate the severity of angiographic and hemodynamic compromise in chronic thromboembolic pulmonary hypertension. Chest 1988; 93(6):1180–5.

16. Nicod P, Peterson K, Levine M, et al. Pulmonary angiography in severe chronic pulmonary hypertension. Ann Intern Med 1987;107(4):565–8.

17. Kovacs G, Berghold A, Scheidl S, et al. Pulmonary arterial pressure during rest and exercise in healthy subjects: a systematic review. Eur Respir J 2009; 34(4):888–94.

18. Auger WR, Fedullo PF, Moser KM, et al. Chronic major-vessel thromboembolic pulmonary artery obstruction: appearance at angiography. Radiology 1992;182(2):393–8.

19. Jenkins DP, Madani M, Mayer E, et al. Surgical treatment of chronic thromboembolic pulmonary hypertension. Eur Respir J 2013;41(3):735–42.

20. Jamieson SW, Auger WR, Fedullo PF, et al. Experience and results with 150 pulmonary thromboendarterectomy operations over a 29-month period. J Thorac Cardiovasc Surg 1993;106(1):116–26 [discussion: 26–7].

21. Thistlethwaite PA, Kaneko K, Madani MM, et al. Technique and outcomes of pulmonary endarterectomy surgery. Ann Thorac Cardiovasc Surg 2008;14(5):274–82.

22. Fedullo P, Kerr KM, Kim NH, et al. Chronic thromboembolic pulmonary hypertension. Am J Respir Crit Care Med 2011;183(12):1605–13.

23. Bonderman D, Skoro-Sajer N, Jakowitsch J, et al. Predictors of outcome in chronic thromboembolic pulmonary hypertension. Circulation 2007;115(16): 2153–8.

24. Madani MM, Auger WR, Pretorius V, et al. Pulmonary endarterectomy: recent changes in a single institution's experience of more than 2,700 patients. Ann Thorac Surg 2012;94(1):97–103 [discussion: 103].

25. Mayer E, Jenkins D, Lindner J, et al. Surgical management and outcome of patients with chronic thromboembolic pulmonary hypertension: results from an international prospective registry. J Thorac Cardiovasc Surg 2011;141(3):702–10.

26. Dartevelle P, Fadel E, Mussot S, et al. Chronic thromboembolic pulmonary hypertension. Eur Respir J 2004;23(4):637–48.

27. Thistlethwaite PA, Kemp A, Du L, et al. Outcomes of pulmonary endarterectomy for treatment of extreme thromboembolic pulmonary hypertension. J Thorac Cardiovasc Surg 2006;131(2):307–13.

28. Levinson RM, Shure D, Moser KM. Reperfusion pulmonary edema after pulmonary artery thromboendarterectomy. Am Rev Respir Dis 1986;134(6): 1241–5.

29. Lee KC, Cho YL, Lee SY. Reperfusion pulmonary edema after pulmonary endarterectomy. Acta Anaesthesiol Sin 2001;39(2):97–101.

30. Kerr KM, Auger WR, Marsh JJ, et al. Efficacy of methylprednisolone in preventing lung injury following pulmonary thromboendarterectomy. Chest 2012;141(1):27–35.

31. Taichman DB, Ornelas J, Chung L, et al. Pharmacologic therapy for pulmonary arterial hypertension in adults: CHEST guideline and expert panel report. Chest 2014;146(2):449–75.

32. Stasch JP, Becker EM, Alonso-Alija C, et al. NO-independent regulatory site on soluble guanylate cyclase. Nature 2001;410(6825):212–5.

33. Hoeper MM. Pharmacological therapy for patients with chronic thromboembolic pulmonary hypertension. Eur Respir Rev 2015;24(136):272–82.

34. Galie N, Corris PA, Frost A, et al. Updated treatment algorithm of pulmonary arterial hypertension. J Am Coll Cardiol 2013;62(25 Suppl):D60–72.

35. Gentles TL, Lock JE, Perry SB. High pressure balloon angioplasty for branch pulmonary artery stenosis: early experience. J Am Coll Cardiol 1993;22(3):867–72.

36. Kreutzer J, Landzberg MJ, Preminger TJ, et al. Isolated peripheral pulmonary artery stenoses in the adult. Circulation 1996;93(7):1417–23.

37. Voorburg JA, Cats VM, Buis B, et al. Balloon angioplasty in the treatment of pulmonary hypertension caused by pulmonary embolism. Chest 1988;94(6): 1249–53.

38. Feinstein JA, Goldhaber SZ, Lock JE, et al. Balloon pulmonary angioplasty for treatment of chronic thromboembolic pulmonary hypertension. Circulation 2001;103(1):10–3.

39. Sugimura K, Fukumoto Y, Satoh K, et al. Percutaneous transluminal pulmonary angioplasty markedly improves pulmonary hemodynamics and long-term prognosis in patients with chronic thromboembolic pulmonary hypertension. Circ J 2012; 76(2):485–8.

40. Kataoka M, Inami T, Hayashida K, et al. Percutaneous transluminal pulmonary angioplasty for the treatment of chronic thromboembolic pulmonary hypertension. Circ Cardiovasc Interv 2012;5(6): 756–62.

41. Mizoguchi H, Ogawa A, Munemasa M, et al. Refined balloon pulmonary angioplasty for inoperable patients with chronic thromboembolic pulmonary hypertension. Circ Cardiovasc Interv 2012;5(6): 748–55.

42. Andreassen AK, Ragnarsson A, Gude E, et al. Balloon pulmonary angioplasty in patients with inoperable chronic thromboembolic pulmonary hypertension. Heart 2013;99(19):1415–20.

43. Inami T, Kataoka M, Ando M, et al. A new era of therapeutic strategies for chronic thromboembolic pulmonary hypertension by two different interventional therapies; pulmonary endarterectomy and percutaneous transluminal pulmonary angioplasty. PLoS One 2014;9(4):e94587.

44. Taniguchi Y, Miyagawa K, Nakayama K, et al. Balloon pulmonary angioplasty: an additional treatment option to improve the prognosis of

patients with chronic thromboembolic pulmonary hypertension. EuroIntervention 2014;10(4):518–25.

45. Inami T, Kataoka M, Yanagisawa R, et al. Long-term outcomes after percutaneous transluminal pulmonary angioplasty for chronic thromboembolic pulmonary hypertension. Circulation 2016;134(24):2030–2.

46. Olsson KM, Wiedenroth CB, Kamp JC, et al. Balloon pulmonary angioplasty for inoperable patients with chronic thromboembolic pulmonary hypertension: the initial German experience. Eur Respir J 2017;49(6) [pii:1602409].

47. Shimura N, Kataoka M, Inami T, et al. Additional percutaneous transluminal pulmonary angioplasty for residual or recurrent pulmonary hypertension after pulmonary endarterectomy. Int J Cardiol 2015;183:138–42.

48. Tsuji A, Ogo T, Demachi J, et al. Rescue balloon pulmonary angioplasty in a rapidly deteriorating chronic thromboembolic pulmonary hypertension patient with liver failure and refractory infection. Pulm Circ 2014;4(1):142–7.

49. Nakamura M, Sunagawa O, Tsuchiya H, et al. Rescue balloon pulmonary angioplasty under veno-arterial extracorporeal membrane oxygenation in a patient with acute exacerbation of chronic thromboembolic pulmonary hypertension. Int Heart J 2015;56(1):116–20.

50. Wiedenroth CB, Liebetrau C, Breithecker A, et al. Combined pulmonary endarterectomy and balloon pulmonary angioplasty in patients with chronic thromboembolic pulmonary hypertension. J Heart Lung Transplant 2016;35(5):591–6.

51. Tatebe S, Fukumoto Y, Sugimura K, et al. Optical coherence tomography as a novel diagnostic tool for distal type chronic thromboembolic pulmonary hypertension. Circ J 2010;74(8):1742–4.

52. Ogo T. Balloon pulmonary angioplasty for inoperable chronic thromboembolic pulmonary hypertension. Curr Opin Pulm Med 2015;21(5):425–31.

53. Tatebe S, Fukumoto Y, Sugimura K, et al. Optical coherence tomography is superior to intravascular ultrasound for diagnosis of distal-type chronic thromboembolic pulmonary hypertension. Circ J 2013;77(4):1081–3.

54. Nair A, Margolis MP, Kuban BD, et al. Automated coronary plaque characterisation with intravascular ultrasound backscatter: ex vivo validation. EuroIntervention 2007;3(1):113–20.

55. Kopec G, Waligora M, Stepniewski J, et al. In vivo characterization of changes in composition of organized thrombus in patient with chronic thromboembolic pulmonary hypertension treated with balloon pulmonary angioplasty. Int J Cardiol 2015;186:279–81.

56. Sugiyama M, Fukuda T, Sanda Y, et al. Organized thrombus in pulmonary arteries in patients with chronic thromboembolic pulmonary hypertension; imaging with cone beam computed tomography. Jpn J Radiol 2014;32(7):375–82.

57. Inami T, Kataoka M, Shimura N, et al. Pressure-wire-guided percutaneous transluminal pulmonary angioplasty: a breakthrough in catheter-interventional therapy for chronic thromboembolic pulmonary hypertension. JACC Cardiovasc Interv 2014;7(11):1297–306.

58. Takei M, Kataoka M, Kawakami T, et al. Underdeveloped bronchial arteries as a risk factor for complications in balloon pulmonary angioplasty. Int J Cardiol 2016;203:1016–7.

59. Inami T, Kataoka M, Shimura N, et al. Pulmonary edema predictive scoring index (PEPSI), a new index to predict risk of reperfusion pulmonary edema and improvement of hemodynamics in percutaneous transluminal pulmonary angioplasty. JACC Cardiovasc Interv 2013;6(7):725–36.

60. Fukui S, Ogo T, Morita Y, et al. Right ventricular reverse remodelling after balloon pulmonary angioplasty. Eur Respir J 2014;43(5):1394–402.

61. Hosokawa K, Abe K, Oi K, et al. Balloon pulmonary angioplasty-related complications and therapeutic strategy in patients with chronic thromboembolic pulmonary hypertension. Int J Cardiol 2015;197:224–6.

62. Fukui S, Ogo T, Goto Y, et al. Exercise intolerance and ventilatory inefficiency improve early after balloon pulmonary angioplasty in patients with inoperable chronic thromboembolic pulmonary hypertension. Int J Cardiol 2015;180:66–8.

63. Hosokawa K, Abe K, Oi K, et al. Negative acute hemodynamic response to balloon pulmonary angioplasty does not predicate the long-term outcome in patients with chronic thromboembolic pulmonary hypertension. Int J Cardiol 2015;188:81–3.

64. Darocha S, Pietura R, Pietrasik A, et al. Improvement in quality of life and hemodynamics in chronic thromboembolic pulmonary hypertension treated with balloon pulmonary angioplasty. Circ J 2017;81:552–7.

65. Tsugu T, Murata M, Kawakami T, et al. Significance of echocardiographic assessment for right ventricular function after balloon pulmonary angioplasty in patients with chronic thromboembolic induced pulmonary hypertension. Am J Cardiol 2015;115(2):256–61.

66. Broch K, Murbraech K, Ragnarsson A, et al. Echocardiographic evidence of right ventricular functional improvement after balloon pulmonary angioplasty in chronic thromboembolic pulmonary hypertension. J Heart Lung Transplant 2016;35(1):80–6.

67. Kimura M, Kohno T, Kawakami T, et al. Balloon pulmonary angioplasty attenuates ongoing myocardial damage in patients with chronic thromboembolic pulmonary hypertension. Int J Cardiol 2016;207:387–9.

68. Kimura M, Kataoka M, Kawakami T, et al. Balloon pulmonary angioplasty using contrast agents improves impaired renal function in patients with chronic thromboembolic pulmonary hypertension. Int J Cardiol 2015;188:41–2.

69. Inami T, Kataoka M, Ishiguro H, et al. Percutaneous transluminal pulmonary angioplasty for chronic thromboembolic pulmonary hypertension with severe right heart failure. Am J Respir Crit Care Med 2014;189(11):1437–9.

70. Yanagisawa R, Kataoka M, Inami T, et al. Safety and efficacy of percutaneous transluminal pulmonary angioplasty in elderly patients. Int J Cardiol 2014;175(2):285–9.

Mechanical Circulatory Support for High-Risk Pulmonary Embolism

Mahir Elder, MD[a],*, Nimrod Blank, MD[a],
Adi Shemesh, MD[a], Mohit Pahuja, MD[a], Amir Kaki, MD[a],
Tamam Mohamad, MD[a], Theodore Schreiber, MD[a],
Jay Giri, MD, MPH[b]

KEYWORDS

- Mechanical circulatory support • Right ventricular failure • Cardiogenic shock
- Pulmonary embolism

KEY POINTS

- Temporary mechanical circulatory support (MCS) devices have a role in treating high-risk patients with pulmonary embolism (PE) with cardiogenic shock.
- Mechanical circulatory device selection should be made based on center experience and device-specific features.
- All current devices are effective in decreasing right atrial pressure and providing circulatory support of 4 to 5 L/min.
- The pulmonary artery pulsatility index may prove to be an unreliable method to assess right ventricular function in high-risk patients with PE with cardiogenic shock.
- Careful clinical evaluation on an individual patient basis should determine the need for MCS.

Venous thromboembolism (VTE) is responsible for the hospitalization of more than 250,000 Americans annually and represents a significant risk for morbidity and mortality. The incidence of pulmonary embolism (PE) is approximately 60 to 70 per 100,000 people.[1] Mortality rates for patients with acute PE may exceed 15% within the first 3 months of presentation.[2]

Acute high-risk (also called "massive") PE is an important cause of acute right ventricular (RV) failure that predisposes to cardiogenic shock and sudden cardiac death. Guidelines for treating acute PE have been published and include treatment guidelines for patients with high-risk PE and cardiogenic shock.[3] However, the evidence base for management of these patients is poor and there is little consensus regarding the

appropriate management for treatment of acute RV failure–induced cardiogenic shock due to PE.

High-risk PE is defined as PE that causes sudden cardiac death or cardiogenic shock (CS) with an associated systolic blood pressure (BP) lower than 90 mm Hg or the need for vasopressor support. In its most severe form, high-risk PE can present as continuous hypotension, profound bradycardia, or pulselessness. Intermediate-risk (also termed "submassive") PE is characterized by evidence of RV dysfunction or myocardial necrosis in the presence of systemic normotension. Other characteristics of intermediate-risk PE are RV strain and the elevation of cardiac markers.[4]

Evaluation of RV function is complex and requires a multimodality approach, including clinical assessment, laboratory studies such as

---

Disclosures: No authors have disclosures relevant to this article.
[a] Department of Medicine, Detroit Medical Center, Wayne State University, 4160 John R Street, Suite 510, Detroit, MI 48201, USA; [b] Division of Cardiovascular Medicine, Penn Cardiovascular Outcomes, Quality and Evaluative Research Center, 3400 Civic Center Boulevard, Philadelphia, PA 19104, USA
* Corresponding author.
E-mail address: melder@dmc.org

Intervent Cardiol Clin 7 (2018) 119–128
https://doi.org/10.1016/j.iccl.2017.09.002

brain natriuretic peptide and troponin, echocardiography, computed tomography/MRI, clinical risk scores, and right heart catheterization with hemodynamic measurements.[5,6]

MANAGEMENT OF PULMONARY EMBOLISM

Unfractionated heparin, fondaparinux, and low-molecular-weight heparin, acting as a bridge to vitamin K antagonists or direct oral anticoagulants, are the mainstays of treatment for patients without hemodynamic compromise. Unstable patients may require escalation of treatment over and above isolated anticoagulation therapy. Risk stratification is critical to guide effective PE treatment in the acute phase. Clinical findings at presentation may facilitate assessment of disease and treatment prognosis. Identifying the presence and severity of RV dysfunction from acute pressure overload represents one of the most important factors in an effective PE risk stratification protocol. Early fully therapeutic anticoagulation is the most important therapy in low-risk and intermediate-risk patients with PE to prevent progression to high-risk status.

PULMONARY EMBOLISM SEVERITY INDEX, SIMPLIFIED PULMONARY EMBOLISM SEVERITY INDEX, AND PULMONARY ARTERY PULSATILITY INDEX

Severity indices to predict PE 30-day mortality risk have been established and are used as part of the patient workup and decision making. PE severity index (PESI) is clinically based and represents the most extensively validated score to date.[7] This score accounts for the severity of PE as well as the patient's existing comorbidities. The PESI score uses 11 clinical criteria, including history of heart failure, systolic BP, heart rate, and O2 saturation, to predict 30-day outcomes of patients with PE.

The simplified PESI (sPESI) score, which uses 8 clinical criteria, also has been validated.[8] Risk stratification via circulating biochemical markers, such as natriuretic peptides and cardiac troponin I or T levels, also may be helpful in determining risk for normotensive patients with PE.[9] Combination of the sPESI with troponin testing provides additional prognostic information.[10] The pulmonary artery pulsatility index (PAPI) is another well-established index used to detect RV failure in myocardial infarction and to predict right-sided heart failure after left ventricular assist device (LVAD) implantation.[11] The PAPI is calculated as pulmonary pulse pressure divided by right arterial (RA) pressure.

One of the greater challenges in treating patients with chronically or acutely compromised RV function is to determine and quantify right heart function and predict outcome. The rationale of the PAPI hemodynamic index is to assess RV function by indexing RV systolic function (pulse pressure) to RV preload (mean RA pressure). Although it has been used to predict outcomes in patients with LVAD, there are no data to support the use of PAPI in patients who suffer acute high-risk and intermediate-risk PE. Unlike in chronic RV failure, as is the case in LVAD candidate patients and in acute RV infarction, in acute PE, the RV myocardium is not directly affected. The increase in cardiac biomarkers represents an increase in afterload and RV strain with minimal damage to the myofibrils themselves.[12,13] Thus, the RV may be more capable of generating enough contractility to generate higher pulse pressure compared with patients with chronic RV failure or acute RV infarction.

PAPI is inversely dependent on preload. In the acute PE setting, preload may remain relatively low or mildly increase unless rapid volume expansion therapy is administered. Moreover, even with volume expansion, the amount of increase in preload is difficult to predict, as it depends on multiple, inaccessible factors such as RA/RV compliance and rigidity, the effect of ventricular interdependence, intravascular volume status, and more.[14] Last, in our experience, PAPI is unreliable in patients with Impella RP (discussed subsequently; Abiomed Inc., Danvers, MA) due to altered PA wave forms, which can result in inaccurate PA systolic and diastolic measurements. In a small series of 4 patients from Detroit Medical Center with high-risk PE treated with Impella RP there was poor correlation between PAPI and the patients' clinical status (**Table 1**, Elder M, unpublished data, 2017).

MANAGEMENT OF RIGHT VENTRICULAR FAILURE

The ability of the RV to immediately adapt to the acute increase in afterload associated with high-risk PE is limited, because the non-preconditioned, thin-walled RV is usually unable to generate a mean pulmonary artery pressure higher than 40 mm Hg. An acute increase of RV afterload generates RV strain and dilation which, per the Starling law, generates more contractility until the dilatation is extreme and contractility falls.[15]

Current guidelines for acute RV failure management include saline infusion as the first step, with an emphasis to avoid excessive

Table 1
A series of 4 patients with high-risk PE and cardiogenic shock treated with Impella RP followed by ultrasound-assisted catheter-directed thrombolysis (EKOS) at Detroit Medical Center

Patient	EKOS No.	Impella Days	PEAK TROP	PEAK BNP	PESI	MOD PESI%	PAPI	HR Before	HR After	Admission	BP Before	After
1	1	3	0.023	758	82	1.1	3.06	94	80	149/82/95	91/59/70	179/94/134
2	2	1	0.092	5069	58	8.9	1.66	106	92	155/112/127	99/69/76	173/97/132
3	1	6	0.434	8245	103	8.9	0.56	103	94	96/80/85	86/71/75	125/85/93
4	2	5	6.166	NA	129	8.9	1.15	124	79	93/60/86	87/56/68	150/71/97

Abbreviations: BNP, brain natriuretic peptide; BP, blood pressure; HR, heart rate; MOD, modified; NA, not available; PAPI, pulmonary artery pulsatility index; PESI, pulmonary embolism severity index; TROP, troponin.

volume overload that may result in extreme RV dilatation and precipitous decline in RV performance as well as bowing of the ventricular septum compromising left ventricular (LV) filling.[16,17] Second-line management includes inotropic or vasopressor support, with no specific agent recommended in consensus guidelines. It has been our experience that epinephrine is the optimal initial vasopressor in the unstable patient with PE, given its positive inotropic effects on the RV with concomitant support of the systemic BP. Milrinone has direct positive inotropic effects on the RV with concomitant pulmonary vasodilator properties. Although it can serve as an adjunctive agent in patients with high-risk PE, it is often not an ideal first choice given its systemic vasodilatory effects. Nitric oxide inhalation, which reduces pulmonary vascular bed resistance, may benefit RV function by reducing RV afterload, though there are currently no established data to show definitive improvement in patients with acute PE.[18–20] Mechanical circulatory support (MCS) of the right heart is an evolving option with both traditional extracorporeal membrane oxygenation (ECMO) and isolated RV percutaneous strategies, such as the Impella RP and Protek Duo (CardiacAssist Inc, Pittsburgh, PA).

EXTRACORPOREAL MEMBRANE OXYGENATION

ECMO involves an extracorporeal circuit that uses a semipermeable membrane for gas exchange. Deoxygenated blood is withdrawn through a drainage ("inflow") cannula by an external continuous flow centrifugal pump, passes through the oxygenator, and is returned to the patient through an "outflow" cannula. These cannulae can be placed percutaneously or surgically into femoral vessels versus centrally into the inferior vena cava (IVC)/RA and aorta. Operators can choose the sizing of the cannulae, which has an impact on the degree of flow within the system. When blood is drained from a central vein and returned to a central vein, a process known as veno-venous (V-V) ECMO, the device serves to provide gas exchange only. Although this oxygenates blood, V-V ECMO does not provide circulatory support for failing RVs or LVs. When blood is drained from the venous system and pumped into an artery, a process known as veno-arterial (V-A) ECMO, the circuit provides both respiratory and circulatory support. Circulatory support with V-A ECMO can exceed 5L per minute. V-A ECMO may increase LV afterload, LV wall tension, and oxygen demand.[21]

Literature regarding ECMO utilization for high-risk PE is scant. A recent systematic review analyzed 78 high-risk PE cases treated with ECMO as described in 19 articles (11 cases reports and 9 case series) that were published over 20 years.[27] Nearly 90% of patients received V-A ECMO and management after initiation of ECMO was variable, ranging from isolated anticoagulation to thrombolysis to surgical embolectomy. The overall in-hospital survival rate was 71% with a 52% survival among the subgroup of 43 patients who had ECMO initiated during cardiac arrest or cardiopulmonary resuscitation. Although mortality in this review was substantial, the predicted mortality rate based on epidemiologic literature ranges from 30% to 80% in the studied population, supporting the concept that the acute stabilization of patients with high-risk PE and refractory shock may be beneficial in properly selected cases.

Technical Perspective for Patients with Pulmonary Embolism

It is relatively unusual for patients with PE to suffer from refractory hypoxemia in the absence of significant hemodynamic compromise. Exceptions to this include patients with severe preexisting lung disease in whom even modest clot burden can result in acute respiratory decompensation or those who experience significant right to left shunting due to a patent foramen ovale. In the latter case, significant RV dysfunction is nearly always present leading to elevated RA pressures and shunting, although the patient may in some cases be able to maintain a stable systemic BP.

Hence, the grand majority of patients experiencing life-threatening PE are suffering from hemodynamic compromise. Thus, V-A, as opposed to V-V, ECMO is the preferred therapy for acute stabilization. The most rapid stabilization is often performed through percutaneous placement of a right common femoral venous inflow cannula (20–22F) with a left common femoral arterial outflow cannula (16–18F). If further right-sided decompression is desired, a second right internal jugular venous inflow cannula can be placed nonemergently (Fig. 1).

Patients undergoing placement of V-A ECMO, especially in emergent situations, are at high risk of major vascular or bleeding complications. This is most commonly from damage to the iliofemoral circulation from the large-bore arterial outflow cannula or direct obstruction of arterial flow to the distal lower extremity. The latter issue can be mitigated through placement

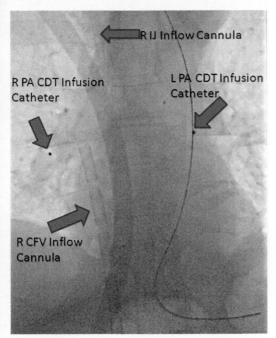

Fig. 1. Fluoroscopy of V-A ECMO in a patient with high-risk PE being treated with catheter-directed thrombolysis.

of an antegrade arterial sheath (5-7F) into the superficial femoral artery that provides perfusion to the limb with the outflow cannula (**Fig. 2**).

Several additional issues arise with V-A ECMO, including an increased incidence of stroke that can be due to embolic phenomena or cerebral hypoperfusion. In patients with a femoral arterial outflow cannula, the oxygenated, re-infused blood may not reach the aortic arch, resulting in suboptimal cerebral or coronary perfusion. Some operators add an additional internal jugular venous outflow cannula to patients in whom this is a concern.[22] This configuration of venous drainage combined with both arterial and venous return (veno-arterial-venous ECMO) may facilitate oxygenation of the cerebral and coronary circulation by returning oxygenated blood directly into the native cardiac circulation while providing circulatory support. The effectiveness of this strategy in a patient with severe RV dysfunction is unknown and is likely to be dependent on the degree of native cardiac stroke volume that the patient is able to produce.

V-A ECMO may increase LV afterload, LV wall tension, and oxygen demand.[23] In the patient who has evidence of significant LV dysfunction, care must be taken to monitor for LV ballooning and worsening dysfunction due to the changes in stress and afterload the LV faces on ECMO. Although there are a variety of techniques for venting (decompressing) the LV in these cases,

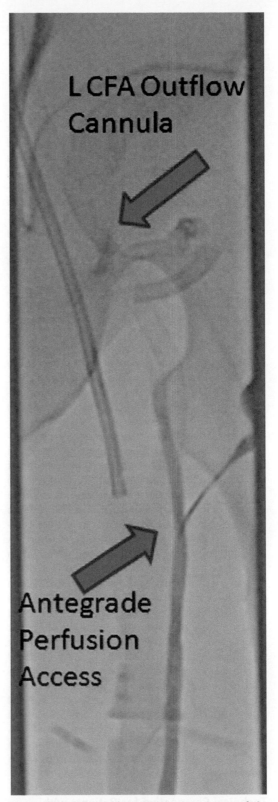

Fig. 2. Fluoroscopy of antegrade cannulation of the left superficial femoral artery to enable limb perfusion in a high-risk patient with PE on V-A ECMO with a left common femoral artery outflow cannula.

this issue is unusual in patients presenting with acute PE as these patients are not generally experiencing an acute LV insult.

IMPELLA RP

In 2015, the Impella RP circulatory support device became the first percutaneous RV support device to be approved by the US Food and Drug Administration (FDA). The Impella RP is a percutaneous, single vascular access axial pump designed for isolated right heart support. The Impella RP heart pump delivers blood from the inlet area, which sits in the IVC, through the cannula to the outlet opening near the tip of the catheter in the pulmonary artery. The device requires a single 23F access into the common femoral vein which is currently the only possible insertion site. The device is advanced into position with its distal outflow in the main pulmonary artery and the proximal inflow in the IVC over a 0.018-inch wire (**Fig. 3**). The device propels blood from the IVC into the pulmonary artery, thus bypassing the RV.[24] The device is able to supply greater than 4.0 L/min output and requires anticoagulation with a target activated clotting time (ACT) of *160 to 180* seconds.[23]

The Recover Right clinical trial,[24] a prospective, multicenter, single-arm study was designed to evaluate the safety and probable benefit of the Impella RP in patients with RV failure (RVF) refractory to medical treatment and deemed to require hemodynamic support. The 30 patients enrolled in the RECOVER RIGHT trial were categorized into 2 patient cohorts. Cohort A included patients who developed RVF within 48 hours after implantation of an LVAD. Cohort B examined patients who developed RVF within 48 hours of postcardiotomy shock or post–acute myocardial infarction shock. It should be noted that high-risk patients with acute PE were not included in this study. The primary endpoint was patient survival at 30 days, hospital discharge, or bridge to the next therapy. Overall, the survival rate was 73% in the entire population at 30 days. Cohort A showed a survival rate of 83.3% and Cohort B had a 58.3% survival rate at 30 days. The study led to conditional FDA approval of the device with the expectation that further post-marketing studies would be conducted.

Technical Perspective for Patients with Pulmonary Embolism

Several issues arise with use of the Impella RP in high-risk patients with acute PE. First, the device

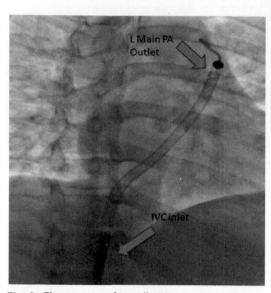

Fig. 3. Fluoroscopy of Impella RP.

provides circulatory support but does not have an oxygenator. Hence, in those patients in whom concomitant hypoxemia is an important consideration, this device is not optimal. Additionally, in patients with associated LV dysfunction, it should be noted that the Impella RP will not provide any LV support and may have unpredictable effects on LV filling pressures. One can consider additional placement of a left-sided Impella device via the arterial system, although this "Bipella" approach is not well studied and does place the patient at risk for some of the same vascular and bleeding complications as that encountered with traditional V-A ECMO.

Most importantly, the anatomy of the PE in the lung must be assessed before placement of the Impella RP. The specific concern that arises is placement of the outflow cannula into a clotted left main PA. This raises the possibility of poor flows through the device or potentially even worsening of the afterload that the RV is facing if the outflow cannula is meeting significant resistance to flow from acute PE. Additional less common concerns include placement of the device in a patient with IVC thrombus that could be sucked into the device.

If the decision is made to place the Impella RP, careful manipulation through the RA and RV outflow tract (RVOT) is necessary. There can be a tendency for this large device to fall apically into the RV rather than track into the RVOT in the patient with a dilated RV.

Although no publications exist with its use in patients with acute PE, several operators have anecdotally used the device to stabilize patients in this setting. At the Detroit Medical Center, we recently used the device to successfully stabilize 4 patients experiencing hypotension with high-risk PE (unpublished data). In all of these cases, we performed ultrasound-assisted catheter-directed lysis after acute hemodynamic stabilization with the Impella RP. Acute hemodynamic profiles and other relevant information about these cases are listed in **Table 1**. All patients survived to discharge.

TandemHeart-ProtekDuo

TandemHeart (Cardiac Assist, Inc, Pittsburgh, PA) is an extracorporeal continuous flow centrifugal pump for temporary circulatory support that can provide up to 8 L/min of flow. TandemHeart support may be V-V, with separate cannulation of jugular and femoral veins, V-A, via peripheral venous and arterial cannulation (15 or 17 Fr), or left atrium-arterial using transseptal 21-Fr cannula to decrease LV filling pressures and afterload and, thus, to prevent LV distension and pulmonary edema and dramatically decrease LV myocardial tension and oxygen consumption.[21] The latter approach is used in cases of isolated LV failure.

The novel ProtekDuo (Cardiac Assist, Inc, Pittsburgh, PA) cannula offers the advantage of minimally invasive percutaneous full right heart support. The ProtekDuo cannula is a flexible, dual-lumen and partially wire-reinforced cannula providing drainage of venous blood through an outer 29-Fr lumen from the RA with output through the tip of an inner 16-Fr cannula into the pulmonary artery, with optional pulmonary support through the addition of an oxygenator into the circuit. The first use of the ProtekDuo cannula/TandemHeart system was performed in Houston, Texas, Memorial Hermann Hospital, in a long-term patient with an LVAD with right heart failure as a bridge to RV adjustment to LVAD.[25]

The ProtekDuo cannula and TandemHeart pump are approved for clinical use for a period of up to 30 days by the European Medicines Agency and up to 6 days by the FDA. Use of the ProtekDuo in cases of high-risk PE have not yet been reported in the literature, although personal correspondence with various operators around the United States indicates that it has anecdotally been used off-label for this purpose in limited fashion.

Technical Perspective for Patients with Pulmonary Embolism
The ProtekDuo provides isolated RV support and also can provide respiratory support through attachment of the optional oxygenator

to the circuit. This makes ProtekDuo a theoretic option for patients who are suffering isolated right heart failure with concomitant severe hypoxemia. The device is very large bore (29F) and is inserted through the right internal jugular vein. A balloon-tipped catheter is used to introduce a 0.035-inch stiff Lunderquist wire (Cook Medical Inc, Bloomington, IN) into the right or left pulmonary artery. The balloon-tipped catheter is then exchanged for the curved ProtekDuo cannula (after serial dilation of the tissue tract in the neck), which has a distal tip that sits in the main pulmonary artery trunk. The placement of the device in the neck allows for the mobilization of the patient, which may be associated with less deconditioning. The manufacturer makes a specially designed vest to facilitate this.

As with the Impella RP, careful assessment of the patient's clot burden is needed before placement of this device. Significant clot burden in the main pulmonary artery or clot-in-transit in the RA could be associated with device malfunctioning or complications. Also, similar to the Impella RP, no published data exist on the use of this device in patients with acute PE.

Similar to a traditional ECMO circuit, the centrifugal pump needs to be primed by evacuating air from the system. Cannulation requires clamping of the connecting tubes and the distal ends of the inflow and outflow cannulae before connecting the tubes. Most centers also require a perfusion specialist to manage the centrifugal pump and oxygenator.

INDICATIONS TO USE MECHANICAL CIRCULATORY SUPPORT FOR PULMONARY EMBOLISM

MCS should be strongly considered in patients with PE with refractory shock or active cardiac arrest. Refractory shock is characterized by the inability to stabilize the patient hemodynamically with modest doses of vasopressors or inotropes. If the hemodynamic status of an patient with acute PE is rapidly changing, consideration should be given to institution of MCS. Other supportive criteria include biochemical signs of end-organ dysfunction, such as an increased serum lactate, blood urea nitrogen, creatinine, or liver function enzymes. When considering this group of patients for MCS, assessment of overall comorbidities and the likelihood of recovery with more definitive PE treatment must be undertaken. Patients with PE often suffer from significant comorbidities that may complicate recovery from the combination of high-risk PE with MCS. At the Hospital of the University

Table 2
Comparison of mechanical circulatory support platforms for high-risk pulmonary embolism

Characteristic	Impella RP	Tandem Heart Protek	V-A ECMO (CentriMag)
Mechanism	Micro-axial	Centrifugal	Centrifugal
Cannula size	24F Peel away, 9-Fr catheter	29–31-Fr dual lumen	14–16 Fr arterial 18–21 Fr venous
Insertion technique	Single femoral vein, 9-Fr catheter remains in vein	Dual-lumen IJ	Peripheral or central
Hemodynamic support	>4 L/min maximum flow	Up to 5 L/min	5 L/min
Hemodynamic effect	RAP – ↓	RAP – ↓	RAP – ↓
	Mean PAP – ↑	Mean PAP –↑	Mean PAP – ↓/No change
	PCWP – ↑	PCWP – ↑	PCWP – ↓
	LV afterload - No change	LV afterload - No change	LV afterload – ↑↑
	Cardiac output - ↑	Cardiac output - ↑	Cardiac output – No change/↓
Implantation time	+	+++	++
Device preparation time	+	++	+++
Anticoagulation	++	+++	++
Postimplant management	+	++	+++
Hemolysis risk	++	++	+
Respiratory support	No	Yes	Yes
Cost	$$	$$$$	$$$
Duration of use	Days	Months	Weeks
Pros	Single access site BiVAD possible with escalation	Ambulate (neck)	Hemodynamic support Oxygenation +++
Cons	No intrinsic oxygenator	Long insertion time, high transfusion rates, transseptal (LA-FA bypass)	LV distension, vascular complications, SIRS Transfusion (bleed) 23Fr

Abbreviations: +, indicate greater; ↑↓ arrows, indicate change from baseline after placement of device; $, indicate cost; BiVAD, bi-ventricular assist device; ECMO, extracorporeal membrane oxygenation; IJ, internal jugular vein; LA-FA, left atrium-femoral artery; LV, left ventricle; PAP, pulmonary artery pressure; PCWP, pulmonary capillary wedge pressure; RAP, right arterial pressure; SIRS, systemic inflammatory response syndrome; V-A, venous-arterial.

of Pennsylvania, for example, we do not offer MCS to patients with PE with metastatic malignancies or those older than 80.

For patients in cardiac arrest, decision making is even more challenging. Often, the cause of the arrest is unknown. At the Hospital of the University of Pennsylvania, we offer immediate mechanical circulation with V-A ECMO to patients with in-hospital arrests that do not carry other life-threatening comorbidities. Patients presenting to the hospital after suffering out-of-hospital cardiac arrest represent a more difficult population given the frequent uncertainty regarding their neurologic status and prognosis for recovery. In these instances, we attempt to evaluate each clinical scenario on a case-by-case basis.

If the decision is made to institute MCS, it is our contention that this is best performed urgently and before any thrombolytic therapy is given when possible. Once a patient is on a stable MCS platform, time can be taken to assess the optimal next steps for more definitive treatment of the high-risk PE. Currently, the most common therapy used in our centers after MCS initiation is catheter-directed thrombolysis. However, we have had patients treated with a range of therapies from isolated anticoagulation to surgical embolectomy after initial stabilization. Given the dearth of comparative data in this area, decision making is undertaken by a multidisciplinary institutional PE response team. The institution of MCS allows for a bridge to decision-making with the patient saved from developing severe and progressive end-organ dysfunction or cardiac arrest while consensus is reached.

In addition to many of the technical issues noted previously, several general issues arise in patients with PE treated with MCS. Complications include severe bleeding from cannulation sites (1 or 2 large-bore venous, V-V, or V-A sites are required). Bleeding may emerge from the gastrointestinal tract in patients who are critically ill. Recommendations mandate the use of heparin for ECMO, Impella RP, and TandemHeart. The target ACT ranges from 160 to 200 based on most publications and manufacturer recommendations.[21] For patients with a contraindication to heparin, bivalirudin and fondaparinux may be used. Intracranial hemorrhage is a devastating complication that is often fatal in this population of patients. Severe thrombocytopenia may occur with any of the devices, most likely due to the mechanical destruction of platelets. Hemolysis is a common complication of the use of MCS devices, with mechanical destruction of erythrocytes. However, hemolysis is usually not severe and rarely causes a significant increase in indirect bilirubin in MCS-treated patients. Thus, its clinical significance remains unknown. Most patients require mechanical ventilation and are subject to risks of ventilator-associated complications. It is important to note that induction of anesthesia in these patients before initiation of mechanical circularity support can often be catastrophic, with precipitous drop in systemic afterload leading to acute cardiovascular arrest. Placement of intracardiac or intrapulmonary cannula can result in traumatic injury to cardiac structures or the pulmonary vasculature. Sepsis is one of the most common complications and the most common cause of death in critically ill patients admitted to the intensive care unit. Prolonged mechanical ventilatory support, bladder catheters, central lines, and large-bore devices predispose patients to infection.

DEVICE SELECTION

After assessing a patient's candidacy for MCS, a decision must be made regarding the most appropriate of the 3 platforms (**Table 2**). There are no comparisons between the different MCS devices to determine superiority of one over another. There are also no data regarding RV recovery or of bridging MCS to RV recovery in patients with PE. In many institutions, availability will be the dictating factor for MCS choice as, even in tertiary care centers, there is no universal availability of these novel circulatory support therapies. In many institutions, round-the-clock availability of a perfusion team that may be necessary for ECMO or ProtekDuo does not exist. Assuming availability of all 3 platforms with associated perfusion and critical care resources, a few important considerations should drive the choice. First, it is important to recognize that ECMO has by far the longest history of use in this population with the other 2 devices explicitly not used in patients with PE during their initial FDA evaluations. With this in mind, factors including appropriateness of the required access sites for cannulation and the need for supplemental oxygenation and/or LV support should be accounted for when choosing an MCS platform in acute PE. It should be noted that there are significant learning curves for the whole team with the setup and use of these devices, so repetitive use of a platform will often lead to more efficient treatment. It is important that protocols for MCS initiation, critical care unit monitoring, and MCS decannulation are in place before starting a program for treatment of high-risk PE with MCS.

SUMMARY

Temporary MCS devices have a role in treating high-risk patients with PE with CS. Mechanical circulatory device selection should be made based on center experience and device-specific features. All current devices are effective in decreasing RA pressure and providing circulatory support of 4 to 5 L/min. PAPI may prove to be an unreliable method to assess RV function in high-risk patients with PE with CS. Careful clinical evaluation on an individual patient basis should determine the need for MCS. Patients with a large PE may decompensate rapidly and the setup time for MCS may be lengthy in a time-sensitive scenario. Thus, we suggest early institution of MCS in patients with clinical signs of impending hemodynamic collapse.

REFERENCES

1. Heit JA, Spencer FA, White RH. The epidemiology of venous thromboembolism. J Thromb Thrombolysis 2016;41(1):3–14.

2. Næss IA, Christiansen S, Romundstad P, et al. Incidence and mortality of venous thrombosis: a population based study. J Thromb Haemost 2007;5(4):692–9.

3. Konstantinides S, Torbicki A, Agnelli G, et al. 2014 ESC guidelines on the diagnosis and management of acute pulmonary embolism. Kardiol Pol 2014;72(11):997–1053.

4. Jaff MR, McMurtry MS, Archer SL, et al. Management of massive and submassive pulmonary embolism, iliofemoral deep vein thrombosis, and chronic thromboembolic pulmonary hypertension. Circulation 2011;123(16):1788–830.

5. Greyson CR. Evaluation of right ventricular function. Curr Cardiol Rep 2011;13(3):194–202.

6. Sanchez O. Prognostic value of right ventricular dysfunction in patients with haemodynamically stable pulmonary embolism: a systematic review. Eur Heart J 2008;29(12):1569–77.

7. Chan CM, Woods C, Shorr AF. The validation and reproducibility of the pulmonary embolism severity index. J Thromb Haemost 2010;8(7):1509–14.

8. Jiménez D, Aujesky D, Moores L, et al. Simplification of the pulmonary embolism severity index for prognostication in patients with acute symptomatic pulmonary embolism. Arch Intern Med 2010;170(15):1383–9.

9. Kucher N, Goldhaber SZ. Cardiac biomarkers for risk stratification of patients with acute pulmonary embolism. Circulation 2003;108(18):2191–4.

10. Lankeit M, Jiménez D, Kostrubiec M, et al. Predictive value of the high-sensitivity troponin T assay and the simplified pulmonary embolism severity index in hemodynamically stable patients with acute pulmonary embolism. Circulation 2011;124(24):2716–24.

11. Kang G, Ha R, Banerjee D. Pulmonary artery pulsatility index predicts right ventricular failure after left ventricular assist device implantation. J Heart Lung Transplant 2016;35(1):67–73.

12. Tulevski II, Hirsch A, Sanson B-J, et al. Increased brain natriuretic peptide as a marker for right ventricular dysfunction in acute pulmonary embolism. Thromb Haemost 2001;86(5):1193–6.

13. Konstantinides S, Geibel A, Olschewski M, et al. Importance of cardiac troponins I and T in risk stratification of patients with acute pulmonary embolism. Circulation 2002;106(10):1263–8.

14. Pinsky MR. Assessment of indices of preload and volume responsiveness. Curr Opin Crit Care 2005;11(3):235–9.

15. Gerges C, Skoro-Sajer N, Lang IM. Right ventricle in acute and chronic pulmonary embolism (2013 Grover Conference series). Pulm Circ 2014;4(3):378–86.

16. Mercat A, Diehl J-L, Meyer G, et al. Hemodynamic effects of fluid loading in acute massive pulmonary embolism. Crit Care Med 1999;27(3):540–4.

17. Ghignone M, Girling L, Prewitt R. Volume expansion versus norepinephrine in treatment of a low cardiac output complicating an acute increase in right ventricular afterload in dogs. Anesthesiology 1984;60(2):132–5.

18. Capellier G, Jacques T, Balvay P, et al. Inhaled nitric oxide in patients with pulmonary embolism. Intensive Care Med 1997;23(10):1089–92.

19. Szold O, Khoury W, Biderman P, et al. Inhaled nitric oxide improves pulmonary functions following massive pulmonary embolism. Crit Care 2006;10(1):P59.

20. Yusuff H, Zochios V, Vuylsteke A. Extracorporeal membrane oxygenation in acute massive pulmonary embolism: a systematic review. Perfusion 2015;30(8):611–6.

21. Abnousi F. The evolution of temporary percutaneous mechanical circulatory support devices: a review of the options and evidence in cardiogenic shock. Curr Cardiol Rep 2015;17(6):40.

22. Choi JH, Kim SW, Kim YU, et al. Application of veno-arterial-venous extracorporeal membrane oxygenation in differential hypoxia. Multidiscip Respir Med 2014;9(1):55.

23. Burzotta F, Trani C, Doshi SN, et al. Impella ventricular support in clinical practice: collaborative viewpoint from a European expert user group. Int J Cardiol 2015;201:684–91.

24. Anderson MB, Goldstein J, Milano C, et al. Benefits of a novel percutaneous ventricular assist device for right heart failure: the prospective RECOVER RIGHT study of the Impella RP device. J Heart Lung Transplant 2015;34(12):1549–60.

25. Kazui T, Tran PL, Echeverria A, et al. Minimally invasive approach for percutaneous CentriMag right ventricular assist device support using a single PROTEKDuo Cannula. J Cardiothorac Surg 2016;11(1):123.

Inferior Vena Cava Filters
Current and Future Concepts

John Andrew Kaufman, MD, MS

KEYWORDS

• Inferior vena cava filter • IVC filter • Caval filter

KEY POINTS

- There is substantial controversy about inferior vena cava filters because of the lack of data supporting effectiveness and increased awareness of complications.
- Overall filter use is decreasing, especially in patients with prophylactic indications.
- Newer devices are being designed to address concerns about low retrieval rates and long-term complications of the devices.

INTRODUCTION

Interruption of the inferior vena cava (IVC) to prevent pulmonary embolism (PE) has been successfully performed since at least 1910, when Fredrick Trendelenburg,[1] MD ligated the IVC of a patient with postpartum septic pelvic thrombophlebitis. Caval interruption to prevent PE did not become widely available or applied until the development of successful intravascular devices, IVC filters, in the 1970s.[2,3] The first generation of IVC filters was designed to be placed through surgical exposure of the femoral or jugular veins because of the large size of the introducers. The clinical utilization of IVC filters subsequently increased as the development of percutaneous insertion techniques and smaller introducers decreased the risk and complexity of the procedure, allowing practitioners without surgical skills to place the devices.[4] Utilization increased in both patients with documented venous thromboembolism (VTE) and those without but who were considered at risk of PE.[4] With the Food and Drug Administration (FDA) approval of the first retrievable IVC filters in 2003, utilization increased dramatically.[5] However, this increase was associated with a relaxation of indications, low rates of retrieval of implanted devices, increased reports of IVC filter–related complications, and the filing of major lawsuits against manufacturers of these devices.[6–9] In 2010 the FDA issued an advisory urging removal of retrievable IVC filters and in 2012 Medicare reimbursement for filter placement was lowered, events that coincided with an observed decrease in IVC filter placements.[10,11] Currently, the use of IVC filters in almost any situation is being questioned in the absence of large randomized clinical trials proving efficacy or benefit but large numbers of publications stressing complications of the devices.[12]

In this review, major trends impacting IVC filters are discussed, including changes in utilization, skepticism about the clinical benefit of filters in general, efforts to increase removal of retrievable devices, and new devices that are designed to meet still-unmet needs and address concerns with current devices. This list is not an exhaustive list of topics related to IVC filters but rather a selection of those that reflect some of the major themes of interest to the medical community and the public.

NOMENCLATURE

Vena cava filters are described using many terms, some of which can confuse the conversation. In this review, the following terms are

Disclosure Statement: Ownership interest, Bio2 Medical; medical board member, Argon Medical; research, consulting, and speaking, Cook Medical.

Department of Interventional Radiology, Dotter Interventional Institute, Oregon Health & Science University, 3181 SW Sam Jackson Park Road, Mail Code L-605, Portland, OR 97239, USA

E-mail address: kaufmajo@ohsu.edu

used: *permanent* indicates a filter that was not designed to be removed; *retrievable* indicates a filter that was designed to be removed using percutaneous techniques but can remain permanently; *convertible* indicates a filter that was designed to remain in place but has the capability of opening so that trapping of emboli is no longer possible; lastly, *temporary* indicates a filter that must be removed, as it is usually tethered to an externalized catheter or wire. In the United States, all retrievable and convertible filters are approved by the FDA as permanent implants. The one temporary filter is approved for a 30-day indwell time.

CHANGES IN UTILIZATION

The United States has always placed disproportionally more IVC filters than any other country and experienced far greater growth in filter utilization.[13] The explanation for this has never been clear, although the observed rate of placement in Medicare patients with PE has remained stable over time even as the absolute number of PE diagnoses has increased.[14] Nationwide, filter utilization varies state by state, and within states from one hospital to another.[15] Nevertheless, filter utilization rates are now decreasing this country, with the inflection point generally accepted as having occurred in 2012.[10,11]

This decrease in utilization overall is appropriate, but there is likely not one explanation for this change. The increased awareness of IVC filter complications has clearly influenced referrals for IVC filter placements. These complications include filter penetration of local structures, filter migration, filter fracture, and embolization of filter fragments to the heart and pulmonary artery circulation.[16] The impact of reporting bias is always speculative; but published IVC filter articles have increasingly focused on complications of the devices, whereas the total number of articles overall has increased dramatically. A simple PubMed search of the terms *IVC filter* and *IVC filter complications* between January 1, 2000 and June 16, 2017 showed that 57% of articles included the term *complications* compared with only 43% of articles between 1985 and 2000. The absolute number of articles on filters increased almost 600% in this same time period. Whether the actual incidence of IVC filter complications has increased or the interest in reporting has increased is not clear. Analyses of the self-reported FDA Manufacturer and User Facility Device Experience (MAUDE) data on device complications demonstrates a disproportion representation of retrievable IVC filters compared with permanent devices and variations between the devices themselves.[7] Unfortunately, the actual denominators are not known, so evidence-based conclusions are difficult.

Over the past 2 decades, one of the drivers of increased filter utilization was the implantation of these devices in patients who did not have VTE but were considered at risk of developing PE and could not have medical prophylaxis (referred to as *prophylactic filters*). The largest group of patients in this category was trauma patients. The use of IVC filters in this patient population in this manner was based on favorable observational series in the 1990s.[17] As data accumulated, the benefits in terms of protection from PE seemed more modest but still positive.[18]

More recently, the benefit of prophylactic IVC filters in this population has been questioned and utilization has decreased.[19,20] Sarosiek and colleagues[20] found no survival benefit in trauma patients receiving IVC filters at a major urban trauma center between 2003 and 2012, with only 8% ultimately being retrieved. In an analysis of several large databases containing 272,391 trauma patients with IVC filters, of which 93% were placed prophylactically, Cook and colleagues[21] found no change in PE rates despite declining utilization of IVC filters between 2003 and 2015. Hemmila and colleagues[19] found no benefit in terms of reduction of mortality but a significantly increased risk of DVT in these patients. The lack of convincing evidence of clinical benefit, the concern that DVT may be increased in patients with filters, and the low retrieval rates haves resulted in decreased utilization of prophylactic filters in trauma patients.

The publicity surrounding IVC filters and their complications increased the awareness of both patients and physicians about the potential complications of these devices. The public is exposed to television advertisements, Internet advertisements, news media reports, and direct mail marketing from law firms stressing the complications from these devices. In this environment, there is a disincentive to recommend IVC filter placement and patients are reluctant to agree to placement.

The utilization of IVC filters has decreased simultaneously with a decrease in reimbursement for the procedure.[11] Whether the change in reimbursement was coincidental with the decline in procedures or causative cannot be determined from the data, but volumes of other procedures have been shown to be correlated with changes in reimbursement.[22] A shift toward a more conservative stance on filters in professional guidelines has also been suggested as a cause for the decrease in filter utilization.[10] Wadhwa and colleagues[23] linked the decrease in utilization to the FDA advisories in 2010. The challenge with all of these hypotheses is the inability to know what is behind the behaviors of the individual providers at the time decisions about filters are made. In all likelihood, the decrease in filter utilization has been multifactorial.

THE DANGER OF SKEPTICISM

The level of uncertainty about IVC filters in the medical community is now extremely high. The current state of knowledge about IVC filters has been called a "data desert," in which there is not enough evidence to justify the use of IVC filters.[12]

There have been only 2 randomized prospective clinical trials of filter efficacy, the Prevention du Risque d'Embolie Pulmonaire par Interruption Cave (PREPIC) I and II trials.[24,25] In both trials, 400 patients with documented VTE who were being anticoagulated were randomized to either a control group (anticoagulation alone) or to receive an additional permanent filter (PREPIC I) or an additional retrievable filter (PREPIC II). The results of PREPIC I suggested that filters provide an early protection from symptomatic recurrent PE but no long-term survival benefit.[25] This finding stimulated the PREPIC II trial in which retrievable filters were used, but the recurrent PE rate was unexpectedly low in the control group. The trial demonstrated that the filter group derived no benefit from the devices and was subjected to more procedures (IVC filter removals).[24] However, both studies were fundamentally flawed in that the populations studied did not have an indication for IVC filtration. All of the patients were eligible for and were treated with anticoagulation, the accepted standard of care. Despite the laudable trial design (randomized, prospective), the data are of very limited utility for guiding practice in many encountered clinical situations.

Population-based retrospective studies have been used in attempts to understand the efficacy of filters. However, analyses of large state and national databases have been contradictory, suggesting both a lack of utility of filters to prevent morbidity and mortality from PE or a modest benefit.[14,26] Although there have been no similar analyses of the impact of

complications of filters, there is widespread concern that these devices may not only have limited (or no) efficacy but could be actually harming patients.[27]

There is no debating the dearth of high-quality data on filters. The risk is that, in the absence of these data, all filters and all indications will be considered suspect, placing some patients at unnecessary risk of PE when devices are withheld. The probability of performing a randomized prospective clinical trial in patients with VTE who cannot be anticoagulated to test the hypothesis that IVC filters prevent morbid and/or lethal PE is low. In a cautious but rational world, these devices should be used in patients who have VTE and cannot be treated with anticoagulation despite the lack of level 1 evidence.

INCREASE IN REMOVALS

The appeal of retrievable IVC filters was based on the concept that they would be removed after the risk of PE became reasonably low.[28] Compared with permanent devices, which remain in place regardless of whether protection from PE is necessary, retrievable devices could be used in a focused manner. The ability to be retrieved did not create new indications for filter placement but rather changed the postprocedure management from passive to active. There is suggestive evidence and a generally accepted notion that filter complications and the difficulty of retrieval increase with time.[29,30] Based on decision analysis modeling, Morales and colleagues[30] recommended IVC filter removal between 29 and 54 days after placement as balancing the risk of PE versus the risk of continued presence of the filter.

The initial reports of retrievals performed outside of clinical trials indicated that retrieval rates were actually very low, especially in trauma patients.[31,32] In response to the observed low rates of retrievals, dedicated IVC filter clinics have been established in many practices. The electronic medical record (EMR) can be an important element in tracking patients with IVC filters and encouraging retrieval when appropriate. Wang and colleagues[33] noted both an increase in IVC filter retrievals and a decrease in IVC filter placements in the Kaiser Health Care system after implementing a physician education program and patient tracking in the EMR. The importance of these clinics and educational efforts is to focus attention on a device that is often placed within the context of a complicated medical or surgical episode and, therefore, easily overlooked in follow-up.

Achieving 100% retrieval is unrealistic, as patient status relative to anticoagulation may change, patients may become lost to follow-up, or patients may choose to keep their filter. In most instances, retrieval rates of filters that were placed with a specific intention to be retrieved can exceed 60% when an organized system for patient follow-up is in place.[34] The importance of systematic follow-up of patients with retrievable IVC filters has been emphasized by adoption of assessment within 3 months for retrieval as a quality metric for the Medicare Accessibility and CHIP Reauthorization Act.[35]

The increased interest in IVC filter retrieval has resulted in an increase in the complexity of the procedures. Filters that are adherent to the wall of the IVC, tilted, fractured, penetrated, and embolized can all be removed percutaneously. Special techniques have been developed for these scenarios, including the application of off-label tools intended for removal of pacemaker leads.[36] Techniques for removing permanent filters have been developed as well.[37] In experienced programs, the success of filter retrieval approaches 95%.[34,38]

The elements of a successful retrieval procedure are careful planning and availability of the necessary tools and skills to complete the procedure. Plain radiography is very useful for confirming the identity of the filter, documenting its integrity, and assessing whether significant tilt or migration has occurred. A preprocedural computed tomography scan (preferably with contrast) should be obtained in any patient with a filter that has been in place for an extended duration (the author uses 6 months) or who has had a prior failed attempt at retrieval.[39] This scan permits careful assessment of the filter in relation to the wall of the IVC and planning for the procedure. Kiefer and colleagues[40] report the value of rotational venography at the time of the procedure, allowing correct identification of tip-imbedded filters compared with anteroposterior venography. During the removal procedure, it is essential to avoid disrupting or distorting a filter unless there is absolute certainty that the filter can be removed. A filter that becomes deranged during a retrieval attempt may no longer provide protection from PE and can lead to complications.[41] Although complications of IVC filter removal are rarely reported, they are likely more prevalent and serious than estimated. In some cases, open removal rather than a percutaneous attempt should be considered.[42]

One of the most glaring inconsistencies regarding opinions about IVC filters is the acceptance of the benefit of removal of these devices. This acceptance prompts very complex and risky procedures and the removal of devices that were never designed to be removed percutaneously.[43] The lack of high-quality data supporting placement of IVC filters is widely accepted. The complete lack of quality data supporting the benefits of IVC filter removal should be acknowledged as well.

NEW DEVICES

The overall decline in IVC filter placements, the negative attitude toward these devices in the medical community and public, the challenges of achieving high rates of filter retrievals, and the increasingly hostile legal environment for manufacturers have greatly influenced the next generation of devices. The value proposition for any new device must be compelling in this ecosystem and able to address some of the major limitations of current devices.

One approach to patients with a short-term risk of PE that addresses the concerns associated with long-term retention of IVC filters and potentially difficult retrievals is a temporary filter (one that is tethered to an externalized catheter and must be removed). The Angel Catheter (Bio2 Medical, Golden, CO) is the only temporary filter that is FDA (August 2016) and Conformité Européenne (CE) (May 2012) approved (**Fig. 1**).[44] Designed for ultrasound-guided bedside placement from a femoral approach in the intensive care or emergency department setting, the device is approved for a 30-day dwell time and can also be used for infusion. Early clinical experience has been encouraging.[45]

A different approach to reducing the need for a second procedure (removal or conversion) and addressing low retrieval rates is a filter that ceases to function as a filter after a specified period of time. The Sentry filter (Novate Medical, Dublin, Ireland) is a permanent device that

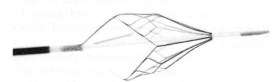

Fig. 1. The Angel Catheter. This filter is the only temporary filter approved in the United States. Designed for percutaneous ultrasound-guided bedside placement through common femoral vein access in critically ill patients, it must be removed by 30 days. (*Courtesy of Bio2 Medical, Golden, CO; with permission.*)

automatically converts from an IVC filter to an open IVC stent at a minimum of 60 days[46] (**Fig. 2**). The mechanism of conversion is a biodegradable filament that holds together the metal filtration elements of the device. When released, these elements retract to the wall of the IVC in a stentlike configuration. The filter was approved by the FDA on February 17, 2017.

A filter that is absorbed completely would also address the issues of the need for a second procedure and low retrieval rates but without a permanent implant. Adient Medical (Pearland, TX) has developed a polydioxanone device that retains filtration integrity for as long as 10 weeks but is ultimately completely absorbed[47] (**Fig. 3**). This device is in first-in-man clinical trials, with a US clinical trial to follow. Both this device and the bio-convertible filter will still require dedicated postplacement follow-up, as the devices will lose their ability to protect patients from PE regardless of patients' clinical or anticoagulation status. Patients who are still at risk of PE at that time of conversion or absorption will need a second device.

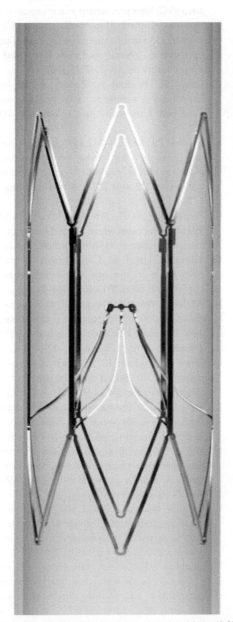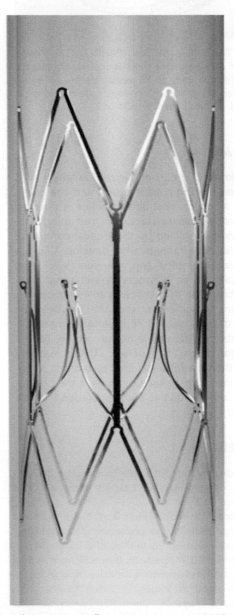

Fig. 2. The Sentry filter is a permanent nitinol-based filter that automatically converts to an open IVC stent at a minimum of 60 days. (*Courtesy of* Novate Medical, Galway, Ireland.)

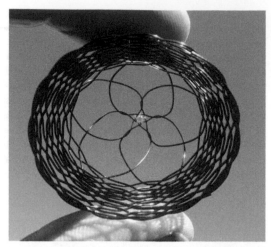

Fig. 3. The Adient Medical (Pearland, TX) filter is made of polydioxanone threads that retain filtration integrity for as long as 10 weeks but are ultimately completely absorbed. (*Courtesy of* Adient Medical, Pearland, TX; with permission.)

SUMMARY

After almost 50 years of clinical availability, IVC filters remain poorly understood and controversial. As a result, most filter practice is directed by opinion rather than fact. This frustrating state of affairs is amplified by the clinical context of these devices. Patients who develop VTE are often very complex and manifest VTE as a complication of or in association with other medical problems. In this confusing environment, it is important to remember that the link between venous thrombosis and PE is certain; when anticoagulation is transiently not an option, IVC filters should be considered. These patients should then be followed in a systematic, organized manner to remove or convert the filter as appropriate as soon as anticoagulation is safely resumed.

REFERENCES

1. Trendelenburg F. Über die chirurgische Behandlung der puerperalen Pyaemie Munchen Med Wschr. 1912.
2. Dodson MG, Mobin-Uddin K, O'Leary JA. Intracaval umbrella-filter for prevention of recurrent pulmonary embolism. South Med J 1971;64(8):1017–8.
3. Greenfield LJ, McCurdy JR, Brown PP, et al. A new intracaval filter permitting continued flow and resolution of emboli. Surgery 1973;73(4):599–606.
4. Stein PD, Kayali F, Olson RE. Twenty-one-year trends in the use of inferior vena cava filters. Arch Intern Med 2004;164(14):1541–5.
5. Yunus TE, Tariq N, Callahan RE, et al. Changes in inferior vena cava filter placement over the past decade at a large community-based academic health center. J Vasc Surg 2008;47(1):157–65.
6. Baadh AS, Zikria JF, Rivoli S, et al. Indications for inferior vena cava filter placement: do physicians comply with guidelines? J Vasc Interv Radiol 2012; 23(8):989–95.
7. Angel LF, Tapson V, Galgon RE, et al. Systematic review of the use of retrievable inferior vena cava filters. J Vasc Interv Radiol 2011;22(11):1522–30.e3.
8. Everhart D, Vaccaro J, Worley K, et al. Retrospective analysis of outcomes following inferior vena cava (IVC) filter placement in a managed care population. J Thromb Thrombolysis 2017;44(2):179–89.
9. Ahmed O, Jilani S, Heussner D, et al. Trapped by controversy: inferior vena cava filters and the law. J Vasc Interv Radiol 2017;28(6):886–8.
10. Desai SS, Naddaf A, Pan J, et al. Impact of consensus statements and reimbursement on vena cava filter utilization. J Vasc Surg 2016;64(2): 425–9.
11. Glocker RJ, TerBush MJ, Hill EL, et al. Bundling of reimbursement for inferior vena cava filter placement resulted in significantly decreased utilization between 2012 and 2014. Ann Vasc Surg 2017;38: 172–6.
12. Bikdeli B, Ross JS, Krumholz HM. Data desert for inferior vena caval filters: limited evidence, supervision, and research. JAMA Cardiol 2017;2(1):3–4.
13. Wang SL, Lloyd AJ. Clinical review: inferior vena cava filters in the age of patient-centered outcomes. Ann Med 2013;45(7):474–81.
14. Bikdeli B, Wang Y, Minges KE, et al. Vena caval filter utilization and outcomes in pulmonary embolism: Medicare hospitalizations from 1999 to 2010. J Am Coll Cardiol 2016;67(9):1027–35.
15. Brown JD, Talbert JC. Variation in the use of vena cava filters for venous thromboembolism in hospitals in Kentucky. JAMA Surg 2016;151(10):984–6.
16. Trerotola SO, Stavropoulos SW. Management of fractured inferior vena cava filters: outcomes by fragment location. Radiology 2017;284(3):887–96.
17. Rogers FB, Strindberg G, Shackford SR, et al. Five-year follow-up of prophylactic vena cava filters in high-risk trauma patients. Arch Surg 1998;133(4): 406–11 [discussion: 412].
18. Haut ER, Garcia LJ, Shihab HM, et al. The effectiveness of prophylactic inferior vena cava filters in trauma patients: a systematic review and meta-analysis. JAMA Surg 2014;149(2):194–202.
19. Hemmila MR, Osborne NH, Henke PK, et al. Prophylactic inferior vena cava filter placement does not result in a survival benefit for trauma patients. Ann Surg 2015;262(4):577–85.
20. Sarosiek S, Rybin D, Weinberg J, et al. Association between inferior vena cava filter insertion in trauma

patients and in-hospital and overall mortality. JAMA Surg 2017;152(1):75–81.

21. Cook AD, Gross BW, Osler TM, et al. Vena cava filter use in trauma and rates of pulmonary embolism, 2003-2015. JAMA Surg 2017;152(8):724–32.

22. Clemens J, Gottlieb JD. Do physicians' financial incentives affect medical treatment and patient health? Am Econ Rev 2014;104(4):1320–49.

23. Wadhwa V, Trivedi PS, Chatterjee K, et al. Decreasing utilization of inferior vena cava filters in post-FDA warning era: insights from 2005 to 2014 Nationwide Inpatient Sample. J Am Coll Radiol 2017;14(9):1144–50.

24. Mismetti P, Laporte S, Pellerin O, et al. Effect of a retrievable inferior vena cava filter plus anticoagulation vs anticoagulation alone on risk of recurrent pulmonary embolism: a randomized clinical trial. JAMA 2015;313(16):1627–35.

25. Eight-year follow-up of patients with permanent vena cava filters in the prevention of pulmonary embolism: the PREPIC (Prevention du Risque d'Embolie Pulmonaire par Interruption Cave) randomized study. Circulation 2005;112(3):416–22.

26. Stein PD, Matta F, Keyes DC, et al. Impact of vena cava filters on in-hospital case fatality rate from pulmonary embolism. Am J Med 2012;125(5):478–84.

27. Redberg RF. Medical devices and the FDA approval process: balancing safety and innovation; comment on "prevalence of fracture and fragment embolization of bard retrievable vena cava filters and clinical implications including cardiac perforation and tamponade". Arch Intern Med 2010; 170(20):1831–3.

28. Kaufman JA, Kinney TB, Streiff MB, et al. Guidelines for the use of retrievable and convertible vena cava filters: report from the Society of Interventional Radiology multidisciplinary consensus conference. J Vasc Interv Radiol 2006;17(3):449–59.

29. Wang SL, Siddiqui A, Rosenthal E. Long-term complications of inferior vena cava filters. J Vasc Surg Venous Lymphat Disord 2017;5(1):33–41.

30. Morales JP, Li X, Irony TZ, et al. Decision analysis of retrievable inferior vena cava filters in patients without pulmonary embolism. J Vasc Surg Venous Lymphat Disord 2013;1(4):376–84.

31. Ferguson EJ, Lurie F, Brown M. Low retrieval rates of temporary inferior vena cava filters in trauma patients. Am Surg 2015;81(4):428–9.

32. Minocha J, Idakoji I, Riaz A, et al. Improving inferior vena cava filter retrieval rates: impact of a dedicated inferior vena cava filter clinic. J Vasc Interv Radiol 2010;21(12):1847–51.

33. Wang SL, Cha HH, Lin JR, et al. Impact of physician education and a dedicated inferior vena cava filter tracking system on inferior vena cava filter use and retrieval rates across a large US Health Care Region. J Vasc Interv Radiol 2016;27(5):740–8.

34. Simon TE, Walker PF, Daab LJ, et al. A quality improvement project to improve inferior vena cava filter retrieval. J Vasc Surg Venous Lymphat Disord 2017;5(1):42–6.

35. Radiology, A.C.o. Appropriate assessment of retrievable inferior vena cava (IVC) filters for removal - National Quality Strategy Domain: Effective Care. 2016. Available at: https://www.acr.org/~/media/ACR/Documents/P4P/2017-MIPS/IR/2017_Measure_421_Registry.pdf.

36. Kuo WT, Odegaard JI, Rosenberg JK, et al. Laser-assisted removal of embedded vena cava filters: a 5-year first-in-human study. Chest 2017;151(2): 417–24.

37. Tamrazi A, Wadhwa V, Holly B, et al. Percutaneous retrieval of permanent inferior vena cava filters. Cardiovasc Intervent Radiol 2016;39(4):538–46.

38. Yoon DY, Vavra AK, Eifler AC, et al. Why temporary filters are not removed: clinical predictors in 1,000 consecutive cases. Ann Vasc Surg 2017;42:64–70.

39. Hong S, Park KM, Jeon YS, et al. Can pre-retrieval computed tomography predict the difficult removal of an implementing an inferior vena cava filter? Vasc Specialist Int 2016;32(4):175–9.

40. Kiefer RM, Pandey N, Trerotola SO, et al. The value of rotational venography versus anterior-posterior venography in 100 consecutive IVC filter retrievals. Cardiovasc Intervent Radiol 2016;39(3):394–9.

41. Chou EL, Sgroi MD, Fujitani RM, et al. Complex hybrid suprarenal inferior vena cava filter retrieval. Ann Vasc Surg 2015;29(1):125.e19-22.

42. Manzur M, Ochoa C, Ham SW, et al. Surgical management of perforated inferior vena cava filters. Ann Vasc Surg 2017;42:25–31.

43. Kuo WT, Deso SE, Robertson SW. Vena Tech LGM filter retrieval 16 years after implantation: piecemeal removal by intentional mechanical fracture. J Vasc Interv Radiol 2013;24(11):1731–7.

44. Bio2Medical. Available at: https://bio2medical.com/. Accessed June 18, 2017.

45. Tapson VF, Hazelton JP, Myers J, et al. Evaluation of a device combining an inferior vena cava filter and a central venous catheter for preventing pulmonary embolism among critically ill trauma patients. J Vasc Interv Radiol 2017;28:1248–54.

46. Medical, N. Available at: http://www.seroba-life-sciences.com/novate/. Accessed June 18, 2017.

47. Eggers MD, McArthur MJ, Figueira TA, et al. Pilot in vivo study of an absorbable polydioxanone vena cava filter. J Vasc Surg Venous Lymphat Disord 2015;3(4):409–20.

Moving?

Make sure your subscription moves with you!

To notify us of your new address, find your **Clinics Account Number** (located on your mailing label above your name), and contact customer service at:

Email: journalscustomerservice-usa@elsevier.com

800-654-2452 (subscribers in the U.S. & Canada)
314-447-8871 (subscribers outside of the U.S. & Canada)

Fax number: 314-447-8029

Elsevier Health Sciences Division
Subscription Customer Service
3251 Riverport Lane
Maryland Heights, MO 63043

*To ensure uninterrupted delivery of your subscription, please notify us at least 4 weeks in advance of move.

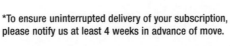

Moving?

Printed and bound by CPI Group (UK) Ltd, Croydon, CR0 4YY

03/10/2024

01040298-0005